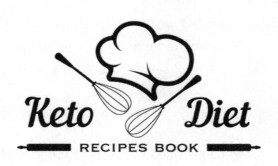

Keto Diet
RECIPES BOOK

KETO AIR FRYER
COOKBOOK FOR BEGINNERS:

Easy and Delicious Ketogenic Diet Recipes
for Weight Loss, Low Carb Healthy Lifestyle
And 4-week meal plan

By Mariah More

Legal Notice:

Disclaimer Notice:

Contents

Detailed
Table of Contents

Chapter 6: Appetizers and Snacks 34

Chapter 7: Poultry Recipes 42

Chapter 8: Beef, Pork and Lamb 54

Chapter 9: Fish and Seafood 64

Chapter 13: Dessert Recipes 96

Conclusion 103

Appendix 1: Measurement Conversion Chart 104

Appendix 2: Air Fryer Cooking Chart 106

Index 107

Introduction

With modern fitness trends, low-carb and high-fat diets are grabbing health fanatics' attention. The keto diet is among these, yet it quite differs from the very popular Paleo, low-carb, and Atkins.

In today's society, easy access to unhealthy food leads to weight gain. Weight gain is one of the world's leading health issues that, in return, leads to several other diseases like diabetes, heart disease, fatty liver disease, indigestion, and many more.

Having access to an abundance of data online to reduce weight and gain health and fitness, people usually feel overwhelmed. They must get authentic context for a particular diet to start following it. Sometimes the diet works, but sometimes it doesn't.

Most people get confused with the idea of high-fat and low-carb, as fat has long been considered something that makes you gain weight. That is incorrect, as cutting sugar rather than fat from the diet has been shown to have many positive effects on health.

High-fat and low-carb help build stamina and more robust muscle, and burn fat, which is what the ketogenic diet is all about.

The ketogenic diet provides good ratios that anyone can follow to reduce weight, regain health, and reduce the symptoms of underlying diseases.

So if you are looking for an excellent diet that reduces weight, and cures recurring health issues like diabetes, cancer, fatty liver, or epilepsy, then this book is just for you.

As you read this book, you will be astonished by the results this diet offers. And to make this healthy transition more successful, we have introduced 1500 days keto diet recipes that are prepared none other than an air fryer. Everyone knows the air fryer is a great kitchen appliance that cooks food in its healthiest form.

If you are not yet familiar with the appliance or keto diet, then worry no more, as this book discusses everything in detail in separate chapters.

Well, talking honestly, for many dieters, the keto diet plan seems very hard at the start, as most of the time, a person may suffer the keto flu, as your body is switching to a new mechanism of burning fats rather than carbs. A genuine commitment to this diet makes everything possible.

Refrain from considering the keto diet a crash diet or a magical elixir that provides results in a shorter time, as it is more than a diet; it's a lifestyle to follow.

Let's start with the basics so that, as a beginner, you get a clear understanding, and then we move forward to the 500 keto air fryer recipes that are delicious and mouthwatering. The recipes also offer snippets of nutrition information to kick-start the keto diet.

So, let's get started.

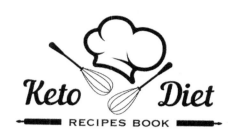

Chapter

1

What Is the Ketogenic Diet Plan?

The keto diet was introduced as an alternative approach to fasting to cure epilepsy. This diet is one of the top-rated diet plans, with many supporting studies and evidence supporting its health benefits. The keto diet plan allows the dieters to consume denser food that satisfies them for extended periods because of the high fat content. A person eats less and gets satisfied, this, in turn, leads to weight loss, better health, and an improved well-being.

The keto diet is all about monitoring what you eat and keeping up with the ratios defined in the diet plan. It is one of the top-followed diet plans as it allows dieters to enjoy their favorite food items like cheese, beef, eggs, and bacon and keep hunger pangs at bay.

If you assume it is a restricted diet plan, we're here to tell you it is not. It is all about adopting healthy habits and eliminating the bad ones.

If you are worried about finding low-carb options, you can easily munch on natural sweets like fruits, dark chocolate, and keto-friendly desserts.

It is not recommended to rush with the diet, as it is necessary to understand and know how it works in order to apply it correctly. The body needs a month to adapt to the new eating system, which helps in weight loss.

The dieter mindset is one of the most significant gaps to overcome. To build stronger muscle, you need to intake more fats in the diet. It helps if you stop treating fat as something bad.

History of the Keto Diet

An endocrinologist named Dr. Rollin introduced the keto diet in 1921, when he studied the ketones produced by the human liver as the result of fasting or when a person eats a high-fat and low-carb diet.

Then, in 1924, Dr. Russell Wilder at Mayo Clinic introduced the keto diet as a plan to treat patients with epilepsy.

It was then that the keto diet turned out to be beneficial for the patients.

But the most important study was done in 1911, when 20 patients were studied while following a vegetarian and keto diet. Only two patients followed the keto diet and showed some astonishing results.

In 1916, Dr. McMurray, based on his studies, found that a low-carb and starch-free diet helps patients suffering from epilepsy.

In 1994, a foundation was created by Charlie Abraham's family named Charlie Foundation after he experienced some of the side effects of the anti-seizure medication he was taking. Then, he followed a low-carb and high-fat diet for five years, which made him seizure-free by the time he reached his college years.

Then, in 1971, Peter Hutten ocher introduced the ketogenic diet. In his introductory diet, 60 percent of the fat comes from MCT oil.

Primary Goal of the Keto Diet

The purpose and essence of the diet are to put the body into a metabolic state that is only achievable by following a low-carb diet. The low-carb diet puts the body in a sugar starvation mood, and as the body needs carbs as fuel, it switches to fat reserves when it finds a lack of carbs and sugar in its diet.

This leads to ketosis, the state in which our body burns fat as an energy source. Results are: better health, weight loss, improved digestion, improved immunity, lowered hypertension, and control of blood sugar.

The keto diet is beneficial in lowering the overall BMI and helps decrease triglycerides, LDL, and bad cholesterol. Moreover, it is a safe diet in the long term.

If you stop consuming fats or lower your fat intake, your body will get into deprivation mode and never feel satisfied or full. This diet offers a ratio that dieters strictly need to follow. The keto diet ratios are given as follows:
- 60-75% of calories from fat
- 5-10% of calories from carbs
- 15-30% of calories from protein

The ratios of the keto diet plan depend on the person's particular needs. Healthy fats like nuts, seeds, olive oil, MCT oil, tofu, lard, and cocoa butter are highly encouraged in the keto diet.

The protein ratio does not discriminate between lean or highly saturated proteins, as the diet encourages you to eat fat like bacon, beef, and pork. Starchy and high-carb fruits and vegetables are discouraged in the keto diet plan. Only certain fruits low in carbs and in a limited proportion are allowed, like strawberries and blueberries. If you want to add vegetables, then go for green leafy vegetables.

Benefits of the Ketogenic Diet
- Improves immunity.
- Lowers anxiety and stress.
- Reduces body inflammation.
- Helps to control and lower the episodes of seizures.
- Helps ease migraines.
- Improves cognitive skills and enhances brain function and memory.
- Helps fight cancer.
- Reduces the symptoms of type 2 diabetes.
- Makes hair stronger and shiny.

- Makes skin glow more.
- Helps reduce weight.
- Improves sleep patterns.
- Assists in GERD control and gallbladder performance.
- Helps prevent gout and maintain a healthy kidney.
- Aids in indigestion by reducing gas and bloating.
- Helps cure fatty liver disease.

Foods That Are Allowed and Foods That Are Not Allowed On the Ketogenic Diet

Foods That Are Allowed. Keto Shopping List

KETO Vegetables: Cabbage, Cucumber, Cauliflower, Broccoli, Broccolini, Asparagus, Radishes, Celery, Green beans, Leafy greens (such as Kale and Spinach), Zucchini, Eggplant, Mushrooms, Kohlrabi, Leek, Garlic, Tomatoes, Jalapeños, Onion, Yellow squash, Spaghetti squash, Bean sprouts, Brussels sprouts, Jicama, Celeriac, Artichokes, Sauerkraut, Kimchi, Peppers, Lemon, Lime, Lettuce

KETO Fruit: Avocados, Blueberries, Raspberries, Strawberries, Blackberries, Kiwifruit, Olives, Rhubarb

KETO Meats: Pork, Beef, Lamb, Goat, Quail, Chicken, Duck, Moose, Venison, Sausages, Wurst, Pâté, Bacon, Prosciutto, Pancetta, Turkey, Jerky, Biltong, Pork rinds

KETO Seafood: Anchovy, Tuna, Herring, Mussels, Oysters, Scallops, Squid, Clams, Shrimp, Octopus, Mackerel, Salmon

KETO Dairy: Cheeses (such as Parmesan, Cheddar, and Gouda, Cream cheese, Mascarpone, and Brie), Heavy Cream, Quark, Greek yogurt, Crème Fraiche, Cottage cheese, Sour cream, Kefir

KETO Dairy Substitutes: Coconut cream/milk, Coconut yogurt, Almond milk, Almond yogurt, Greek yogurt

KETO Nuts: Brazil nuts, Pecans, Almonds, Macadamias, Walnuts, Pili nuts, Pine nuts, Tiger nuts

KETO Seeds: Hemp seeds, Flax seeds, Poppy seeds, Pumpkin seeds, Sesame seeds, Sunflower seeds, Sesame seed paste, and Chia seeds

KETO Fats and Oils: Olive oil, Avocado oil, Butter, Coconut oil, Garlic butter, Ghee, Flaxseed oil, Hemp oil, Tallow, Duck fat, Bacon fat, MCT oil

KETO Sauces: Vinegar, Coconut aminos, Pesto, Mayonnaise, Hot sauce, Guacamole, Creamy dressings, Mustard, Béarnaise sauce, Sesame oil, Low-sugar ketchup, Chipotle sauce, Jalapeño sauce, Worcestershire sauce, Lemon or lime juice, Vinegar-based dressings, Salad dressings, Sugar-free tomato-based sauces, Balsamic vinegar is low in sugar, Wine vinegar, Marinara sauce

KETO Beverages: Low-sugar drinks, Bone broth, Sugar-free syrups, Herbal Tea, Sparkling water (sugarless), Coffee, Dry red wine, Soda water, Dry white wine, Gin, Whiskey, Scotch, Tequila

KETO Cooking Ingredients: Spices, Herbs, Cacao, Almond flour, Peanut flour, Tiger nut flour, Coconut flour, Cacao butter, Stevia, Erythritol, Psyllium husk, Celtic or Himalayan pink salt, Flax meal, Monk fruit, Vanilla extract, Xanthan gum, Dark chocolate, Arrowroot powder

KETO Seasonings for this Recipe Book: Chili powder, Black pepper, Paprika powder, Garlic powder, Ground cayenne pepper, Thyme, Oregano, Cumin powder, Ginger, Curry paste, Coriander powder, Cajun seasoning, Onion powder, Lemon pepper, Italian seasonings, Garam Masala, Poultry seasoning, Dried marjoram, Steak seasoning, Five-spice powder, Dry mustard, Vanilla extract, Cream of tartar, Coconut cream, Old Bay seasoning, Psyllium husk powder, Cinnamon powder, Ground flax seed, Coconut aminos

Foods That Are Not Allowed

Milk and low-fat dairy: cow's milk, rice milk, oat milk, condensed milk, goat's milk, skim milk, skim mozzarella cheese, fat-free yogurt, low-fat cheese, and low-fat cream cheese

Fruit: banana, grapes, mango, plums, grapefruit, oranges, watermelon, peaches, apples, melon, pineapple, pears

Root Vegetables: potatoes (both sweet and regular), carrots, turnips, yams, parsnips, yucca, and beets

Legumes: soybeans, navy beans, black beans, kidney beans, chickpeas, pinto beans, peas, lentils

Grain Products: quinoa, barley, millet, bulgur, amaranth, buckwheat, sprouted grains flour, corn, oatmeal, pizza, popcorn, bread, cereal, pasta, rice, crackers, granola, bagels, muesli

Beverages: beer, apple cider, sweet wines, packaged juice, artificial flavored smoothies, canned sodas

Oils: grapeseed oil, peanut oil, canola oil, sunflower oil, and soybean oil

Sweeteners: honey, cane sugar, maple syrup, agave nectar, Splenda, corn syrup

Sweets: cakes, pastries, pies, candy, chocolate, buns, tarts, ice cream, cookies, pudding, custard, sweetened sauces

Ketogenic Diet and Weight Loss

If you are overweight and tired of following diet plans, it might sound like a marketing gambit to you that the keto diet would be your best choice.

Being overweight is the primary cause of lower self-esteem, anxiety, and depression. It also leads to bloating, gas, indigestion, and gut-related issues, thus leading to high blood pressure and cholesterol.

For all those who find it hard to lose weight, the word "diet" seems depressing to them, as the thought of excluding their favorite food makes it hard for them to kick-start a journey. If you do not like following a restricted diet and do not have the stamina to join a gym, then the keto diet is just for you.

Motivation and commitment are critical factors in making the keto diet successful. When you follow a keto diet, the average weight loss for the first 7 days is 5 to 10 pounds or more, depending on your starting weight. This water weight flushes out the body excessively during the first 14 days of the keto diet. These two weeks are the time in which the body adjusts to the Keto diet. After the first two weeks, the weight loss process slows down but gets a steadier pace.

During the third week, the body gets used to the keto diet and starts burning the fats. Thus, ketosis begins. Ketosis makes a person feel less hungry and more satisfied. It is the most effective way to lose weight.

The acidity caused by ketosis can be flushed out through urine to eliminate its effects; thus, drinking plenty of water is recommended.

How to Identify the State of Ketosis

- The person who follows a keto diet can quickly identify the state of ketosis as the breath changes and starts smelling like nail polish.
- The urge to urinate increases.
- Most people feel nausea, vomiting, stomach pain, and discomfort.
- Once ketosis starts, you feel more tired than usual.
- You may feel confused.

Tips to Lose Weight on the Keto Diet

- Follow the ratios and rules of the keto diet correctly.
- Keep protein intake the same as defined in the keto diet, as a high protein consumption ensures the body turns protein into carbs.
- Eliminate all dairy products like yogurt.
- Drink plenty of water.
- Try intermittent fasting.
- Eat a proper meal and avoid food starvation, as it causes metabolic damage.

The keto diet helps reduce carb intake to 50 grams per day, and fats make up 75 percent of the total calories.

Ketones are produced by the body during ketosis as the carb supply is very limited. Thus the keto diet becomes effective in weight loss and reducing overall body fat percentage.

Suppose you are suffering from a severe underlying issue. In that case, it is crucial to talk to your doctor before starting the keto diet plan, as proper screening by a professional is necessary.

What Is the Keto Flu?

Suppose your sleep is not enough during the keto diet due to stress, hormonal changes, medication, sleep apnea, caffeine use, or consumption of alcohol. In this case, all these conditions can be addressed and cured by taking preventive measures and providing solutions to each problem.

But if your sleep is not disturbed by these factors, you might have the keto flu.

The keto flu is a regular occurrence when the body switches to ketosis.

Keto flu symptoms are the following:

- Stomach pain
- Soreness
- Diarrhea
- Brain fog
- Dizziness
- Instability
- Muscle cramps
- Lack of focus
- Sugar cravings
- Heart palpitations

The keto flu lasts around 72 hours, so insomnia also subsides in parallel. The high-fat and low-carb intakes also temporarily disturb the body's sleep mechanism, as the electrolyte imbalance can lead to a lack of slumber. But it's not a long-term problem, as the sleep issues go away independently.

Some Tips on the Keto Diet to Stay Away from the Keto Flu

- If you eat dinner late, then try eating 2 hours before sleep.
- You can also correct your electrolytes levels by supplement intake; it helps cure insomnia and enables you to sleep much better. Electrolytes also help to relax muscles.
- Turn off regular lights and do not use your mobile; use only blue light before bedtime.
- Exercising or having an active routine is an excellent way to get sleepy and lose weight.
- Try yoga and meditation.
- If you want to enjoy carbs according to the keto ratios for your meal plan, then eat them during the day.
- Avoid coffee or tea before bedtime.
- One factor that needs to be addressed is that when a person starts a keto diet, ketosis puts the body into stress mode. The body is deprived of its current energy source and forced to rely on fats.
- Many people think stress makes a person fat; this is wrong, as stress hormones promote weight loss during stress because they release fat from the body's fat tissues unless it is chronic.

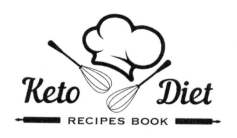

Chapter
2

Getting to Know the Air Fryer

While following a keto diet, you might be experiencing a lot of changes inside you while your body is adjusting to the new mechanism of ketosis. According to the keto diet plan, the most essential hurdle would be easy cooking at home. Keeping all that in mind, we have chosen an air fryer that works with the push of a button. An air fryer is an excellent appliance that offers effortless cooking with energy-saving features.

If you are following a keto diet and managing your busy routine while looking forward to reaping the benefits of weight loss through this diet, then an air fryer is the handiest appliance you will ever have.

An air fryer is a single appliance that can handle several functions simultaneously without hustle. It prepares even the most challenging meat part to its tender perfection. Now enjoy a juicy steak at home and ditch the take-out and restaurant meals to avail the keto diet benefits.

The air fryer is not like a traditional deep fryer. The deep fryer kills the nutrients inside the food, while the air fryer keeps the nutrients intact. The food was cooked, resulting in a crispy food texture.

If you are a beginner, you can use this easy-to-operate appliance for cooking keto-friendly meals that taste great and give your taste buds a delicious ride of flavor. The food we deep fry tastes excellent, but it's full of trans fats and leads to several health issues. The air fryer cooks the food to crispy perfection while keeping the bad fats away. It consumes 80 % less energy, and provides an odor-free and hands-free cooking experience.

An air fryer is a modern appliance that can replace your deep fryers, stoves, and oven and gives you a healthy alternative for your deep-fried items. It simply circulates hot air around the food, making it crunchy and crispy, and satisfying your taste buds as if they were fried items.

Benefits of the Air fryer

- Offers easy maintenance, and it's easy to clean.
- Offers an odor-free and hands-free cooking experience.
- Its operation and function buttons are easy to operate.
- Air fryers have a user-friendly display.
- The air fryer accessories and removable parts are dishwasher-safe.
- Helps you to eat healthily.
- Keeps the nutrients of the food intact.
- You can satisfy your food cravings without weight gain.
- Doesn't heat the atmosphere.
- Cooks frozen food items to tender perfection.

5 Tips for the Air fryer

- It's recommended that you preheat your air fryer before adding food. It saves not only the cooking time but also the meal is prepared much faster.
- If parchment paper is not layered, the air fryer basket or rack gets sticky because of food residues. So, always layer butter paper or parchment paper. Moreover, this also helps to collect the grease without making a mess.
- Fill the rack or basket of the air fryer according to its capacity and never overcrowd it with food.
- Flipping most of the food halfway through for even cooking is recommended.
- The air fryer can be easily opened during cooking without interrupting its cooking cycle.
- Take out the basket, shake it, toss the food, and return it to the air fryer.
- Continuously mist the food with oil spray for a crispy texture.

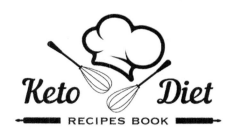

Chapter

3

4 – Week Diet Plan

The 4-week diet plan introduced in this book offers great ideas for recipes throughout each day for a whole month. This 4-week diet plan helps you to focus on your mission to follow a keto diet plan while making it easy to prepare recipes using an air fryer.

WEEK 1					
	Breakfast	Lunch	Dinner	Snack	Dessert
Day 1	Classic Omelet	Wings with Blue Cheese Dressing	Steak and Vegetable	Beef Jerky	Cocoa Cupcake
Day 2	Easy Pancake	Spicy Chicken Breast with Green Beans	Salmon with Coconut	Crab Sticks	Strawberry Shortcake
Day 3	Breakfast Sandwich	Sweet Glazed Salmon	Marinated Lamb Chops	Sausage Bacon Bi	3 Ingredients Cookies
Day 4	Hard Boiled Eggs for Breakfast	Pork Chops	Frozen Fish Fillet with Mayonnaise	Poppers Peppers	Coconut Cookies
Day 5	Green Chili Eggs	Crumbed Chicken Schnitzel	Smoked Salmon	Bacon Wrapped Green Beans	Blueberry Crumble
Day 6	Classic Breakfast Frittata	Salmon with Creamy Dill Sauce	Pesto Salmon	Cheese Puffs	Lemon Biscuits
Day 7	Cheddar Quiche	Veggies Rolls	Sticky Beef Ribs	Mini Pepper Nachos	Pine Nut Cookies

WEEK 2

	Breakfast	Lunch	Dinner	Snack	Dessert
Day 1	Scrambled Pancakes	Pork Meat and Cabbage Rolls	Hearty Lamb Chops Tomatina	Cauliflower tots	Chocolate Cheesecake
Day 2	Breakfast Bacon	Sundried Tomato with Salmon	Cheese-Filled Beef Roll-Ups	Pepperoni Chips	Vanilla Meringues
Day 3	Fluffy Chocolate Chip Pancakes	Spicy Beef Tenderloin	Pesto Salmon	Roasted Purple Cauliflower	Pecans Brownies
Day 4	Roasted Red Pepper and Ricotta Frittata	Spiced Cabbage	Crispy Tofu	Cheese Puffs	Chewy Coconut Biscuits
Day 5	Bacon Egg Muffins	Classic Catfish	Wings with Blue Cheese Dressing	Poppers Peppers	Almond Butter Cookies
Day 6	Easy Pancakes	Glazed Tomato Chicken Kabobs	Salmon with Sauce	Spicy Veggies with Cheese	Chocolate Chip Cookies
Day 7	Classic Omelet	Pork Bites	Zesty Chicken Breasts	Artichokes with Dijon	Lime Macaroons

WEEK 3

	Breakfast	Lunch	Dinner	Snack	Dessert
Day 1	Cottage Cheese Pancakes	Hot Parmesan Chicken Wings	Turkey Patties	Crab Sticks	Pine Nut Cookies
Day 2	Classic Breakfast Frittata	Breaded Sea Scallops	Cauliflower Bites	Cinnamon Nut Scrolls	Simple Cookies
Day 3	Kale Pancakes	Fajita-Stuffed Chicken	Rump Steak	Boneless Wings	Eggless Cake
Day 4	Classic Omelet	Mustard and Rosemary Rib Eye Steak	Cheesy Baked Asparagus	Cheese Filled Mushrooms	Pumpkin Bread
Day 5	Scrambled Pancakes	Greek Roasted Vegetables	Chicken Kabobs with Onions and Bell Peppers	Bacon Wrapped Green Beans	Pecans Brownies
Day 6	Zucchini Egg Cups	Crispy Tofu	Delicious Chicken Sausage Mix	Pepperoni Chips	Cocoa Cupcake
Day 7	Easy Breakfast Sausage	Crumbed Chicken Schnitzel	Rib Eye with Zucchini Noodles	Snack Time Stuffed Zucchini	Apple Cider Vinegar Donuts

WEEK 4

	Breakfast	Lunch	Dinner	Snack	Dessert
Day 1	Breakfast Omelet	Pickle Mayo Chicken Tenders	Sticky Beef Ribs	Roasted Nuts	Chocolate Cake
Day 2	Peanut Butter Porridge	Juicy vegetables and Sirloin Steak with Sour Cream	Pork Meat and Cabbage Rolls	Crab Cake Fritters	Super Moist Cupcake
Day 3	Classic Breakfast Frittata	Salmon with Creamy Dill Sauce	Fish and Okra Stew	Beef Jerky	Almond Butter Cookies
Day 4	Prosciutto and Spinach Egg Cups	Spinach Artichoke Stuffed Peppers	Simple Beef Kebab	Crab Cake Fritters	Simple Chocolate Pudding
Day 5	Cheddar Quiche	Fish Fillet with Onion Rings	Cheesy Eggplant Parmesan	Boneless Wings	Chocolate Cheesecake
Day 6	Jalapeño Bacon Egg Cups	Bourbon Lamb Chops	Crispy Tofu	Bacon-Wrapped Asparagus	Coconut Meringues
Day 7	Breakfast Egg Bites	Avocados with Mayo Sauce	Salmon with Sauce	Simple Tempeh	Blueberry Crumble

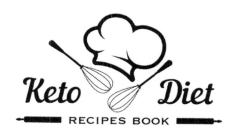

Chapter

4

Breakfast Recipes

— Breakfast Omelet —

Prep: 12 Minutes | Cook Time: 8-10Minutes | Makes: 3 Servings

Ingredients:

- 6 eggs, organic
- 2 tablespoons of butter
- 4 tablespoons of coconut milk
- 4 tablespoons of cheese, grated
- 1 small green onion
- 1 green chili chopped
- 4 tablespoons of red tomatoes, chopped
- Oil Spray, For Greasing, Salt, to taste

Directions:

1. First, preheat the air fryer for 4-6 minutes at 350 ° F(175°C). Meanwhile, whisk eggs, butter, and coconut milk in a large mixing bowl. Dump the grated cheese and whisk it well. Season the egg mixture with salt. Add green onions, chilies, and red tomatoes, and stir.
2. Transfer this egg mixture to an oil-greased cake that fits inside the inside air fryer basket. Once the egg mixture is poured, add the cake pan to the basket.
3. Add the basket to the unit. Close the air fryer. Air fry it for 8-10 minutes at 350 ° F (175°C). Once cooked, serve hot.

Per serving:

Calories 283 | Total Fat 24.5g 31% | Total Carbohydrate 2.6g 1% | Dietary Fiber 0.7g 2% | Protein 14.1g

— Classic Breakfast Frittata —

Prep: 12 Minutes | Cook Time: 12 Minutes | Makes: 3 Servings

Ingredients:

- 6 small eggs, lightly beaten
- ½ pound (225gr) sausage, cooked and crumbled
- ½ cup cheddar cheese, shredded
- 1/3 cup green bell pepper, chopped
- 1/3 of green onion, chopped
- Salt and black pepper, to taste
- 1 teaspoon of olive oil for greasing

Directions:

1. Preheat the air fryer for 6 minutes at 320 ° F (160°C). Take a large bowl and whisk eggs. Next, add crumbled sausages, cheddar cheese, green bell pepper, and green onions. Mix it well
2. Season it with salt and black pepper. Take a heatproof cake pan that fits inside your air fryer basket. Grease the cake pan with olive oil.
3. Transfer the bowl mixture to the greased cake pan. Place the pan into the air fryer basket. Place the basket inside the air fryer. Air fryer it at 370 ° F (190°C) for 12 minutes. Once it's done, serve.

Per serving:

Calories 456 | Total Fat 36.6g 47% | Total Carbohydrate 2g 1% | Dietary Fiber 0.2g 1% | Protein 28.9g

— Breakfast Sandwich —

Prep: 20 Minutes | Cook Time: 15 Minutes | Makes: 4 Servings

Ingredients:
Keto bread Ingredients:
- 4 organic eggs
- 8 teaspoons cream cheese at room temperature
- 4 teaspoons butter, melted
- 1-ounce (30gr) almond flour
- ¾ ounces (22gr) of whey protein isolate
- Salt, to taste
- 1 tablespoon baking soda
- Oil spray for greasing

Ingredients: for Tuna filling:
- ½ cup mayonnaise
- 7 ounces tuna in water, drained
- 2 teaspoons onion powder
- ½ cup celery stalks, finely chopped
- ½ cup pickles, finely chopped (optional)
- Salt and ground black pepper to taste
- 6 ounces (170gr) tomato, sliced
- 4-6 slices of cheddar cheese

Directions:
1. First, preheat the air fryer to 355 ° F(180°C) for a few minutes. Grease a basket of air fryers with parchment paper. Now take a medium bowl, whisk the egg in it, and add cream cheese and melted butter. Mix it well.
2. Then add almond flour, whey protein isolate, salt, and baking soda. Mix it for good incorporation. Add this batter to a loaf pan greased with oil spray and lined with butter paper. Now add all the mixture to the pan and add it to the basket.
3. Add a basket to the unit and close it. Let it bake for 12 minutes at 350 ° F (180°C). Cool down the bread and cut it into squares.
4. Prepare the filling. Take a cake pan and line it with parchment paper.
5. Add mayonnaise, tuna, onion powder, celery, pickles, salt, and black pepper in a bowl. Place this mixture between the bread slices. Top with the sliced tomatoes, tuna mixture, and cheese. Add the other half of the bread on top.
6. Bake in the air fryer for about 3 minutes at 350 ° F (180°C). Serve and enjoy.

Per serving:

Calories 501|Total Fat 36.8g 47%|Total Carbohydrate 14.5g 5%|Dietary Fiber 1.8g 6%|Protein 29.5g

— Classic Omelet —

Prep: 15 Minutes | Cook Time: 8-10 Minutes | Makes: 2 Servings

Ingredients:
- Olive oil spray for greasing
- 4 eggs, whisked
- 2 tablespoons heavy cream
- 2 teaspoons green onion diced
- Salt and black pepper, to taste
- 4 tablespoons of diced Ham
- 4 tablespoons mozzarella cheese shredded

Directions:
1. Preheat the air fryer for 4 minutes at 350 ° F (180°C). Take a round air fryer pan that fits inside the air fryer basket. Grease the air fryer pan with oil spray. Whisk eggs in a bowl.
2. Stir in heavy cream and give it a good mix. Then add green onions, salt, pepper, and diced Ham. Top it with mozzarella cheese. Stir it twice and pour it into an air fryer round pan that fits inside the basket. Sprinkle some additional cheese on top.
3. Place the basket inside the air fryer. Bake it for 8-10 minutes at 350 ° F (180°C) until the cheese melts and the egg is fully set. Serve and enjoy.

Per serving:

Calories 190 | Total Fat 13.7g 18% | Total Carbohydrate 1.7g 1% | Dietary Fiber 0g 0% | Protein 15.5g

— Egg Wrap —

Prep: 10 Minutes | Cook Time: 8 Minutes | Makes: 1 Serving

Ingredients:
- 2 large eggs
- Salt and black pepper, to taste
- ½ teaspoon butter
- 2 teaspoons tomato, pureed
- 4 teaspoons mozzarella cheese, shredded
- 1.5 ounces (40gr) salami, sliced

Directions:
1. Take a small round cake pan and grease it with oil spray. Whisk eggs in a bowl and season it with salt and pepper. Pour the eggs into the cake pan.
2. Add the cake pan to the air fryer basket. Air fry it at 350 ° F (180°C) for 8 minutes.
3. Then take out the cake pan and transfer the omelet to a plate. Top the omelet with butter, tomato puree, cheese, and salami. Roll and serve.

Per serving:

Calories 557 | Total Fat 38.2g 49% | Total Carbohydrate 5.9g 2% | Dietary Fiber 0.2g 1% | Protein 48.3g

— Fried Eggs —

Prep: 10 Minutes | Cook Time: 5 Minutes | Makes: 1 Serving

Ingredients:

- Oil spray for greasing
- 2 large eggs

Directions:

1. Take a pie tin and grease it with oil spray. Now crack eggs into the pie tin and add the pie tin to the air fryer basket.
2. Bake it for 3-5 minutes at 375 ° F (190°C). Five minutes make a runny yolk, so if you want to cook it more, add more time to the cooking cycle.

Per serving:

Calories 126 | Total Fat 8.8g 11% | Total Carbohydrate 0.7g 0% | Dietary Fiber 0g 0% | Protein 11.1g

— Breakfast Egg Bites —

Prep: 12 Minutes | Cook Time: 14 Minutes | Makes: 2 Servings

Ingredients:

- 4 eggs
- 2 teaspoons sour cream
- ½ teaspoon Italian seasoning
- ¼ teaspoon chili powder
- Sea salt and black pepper to taste
- Oil spray for greasing
- 4 ounces (115gr) of Ham or bacon, diced
- 2 cherry tomatoes, quartered
- 2 jalapeno peppers, sliced
- 4 ounces (115gr) of cheddar cheese, shredded
- 2 teaspoons of parsley for topping and chopped

Directions:

1. Preheat the air fryer to 300 ° F (150°C) for 5 minutes. Take a large bowl and whisk eggs in it. Then add and stir in the sour cream.
2. Mix it well, then season it with Italian seasoning, chili powder, salt, and black pepper. Mix it well.
3. Then take ramekins and grease them ramekins with oil spray. Add the equally divided Ham to the bottom of the ramekins, followed by cherry tomatoes and jalapeno slices. Equally, divide the beaten eggs onto each ramekin.
4. Add the ramekins to the air fryer basket. Add the basket to the unit. Air fry at 300 ° F (150°C) for 12 minutes.
5. Then take out the basket and sprinkle cheese on top of the egg ramekin. Air fry for 2 more minutes. Serve with toppings of parsley, and enjoy.

Per serving:

Calories 609 | Total Fat 47.6g 61%| Total Carbohydrate 5.4g 2% | Dietary Fiber 0.8g 3% | Protein 40g

— Scrambled Pancakes —

Prep: 10 Minutes | Cook Time: 9 Minutes | Makes: 1 Serving

Ingredients:

- 2 large organic eggs
- 1/3 cup coconut milk, unsweetened
- 8 teaspoons almond flour
- ½ tablespoon of ground Psyllium husk powder
- ½ tablespoon baking soda
- Salt, just a pinch, 2 teaspoons butter

Directions:

1. Take a large bowl, add eggs and whisk the eggs well. Add coconut milk and almond flour and make pancake batter. Then add Psyllium powder, baking soda, and salt. Melt butter in a microwave and add it to the pancake mix.
2. Take a round cake pan that fits inside the air fryer basket and grease it with oil spray. Pour all the pancake batter into the cake pan.
3. Add into the air fryer and air fry at 350 ° F (180°C) for 4 minutes. Take out the cake pan and scramble the batter, then again air fry for 5 minutes. Once firm, take out the scramble pancake and serve.

Per serving:

Calories 538 | Total Fat 43.3g 55% | Total Carbohydrate 22.2g 8% | Dietary Fiber 9.2g 33% | Protein 17.5g

— Jalapeño Bacon Egg Cups —

Prep: 15 Minutes | Cook Time: 12 Minutes | Makes: 2 Servings

Ingredients:

- 1 cup Mexican blend cheese shredded
- 2 regular jalapeno peppers finely chopped
- 10 tablespoons bacon bits
- 10 large eggs
- 1/3 cup sour cream
- 1 teaspoon garlic powder, Salt and pepper to taste

Directions:

1. Preheat the air fryer for 4 minutes at 350 ° F(180°C). Take 6 (2.5 inches 60mm) ramekins and line them with muffin cups. Distribute cheese, jalapeno, and bacon into each muffin cup.
2. Crack eggs in a bowl and whisk them with sour cream, garlic powder, salt, and pepper. Divide this egg mixture into the ramekins.
3. Add the ramekins to the air fryer and air fry for 12 minutes at 350 ° F (180°C). Once done, serve.

Per serving:

Calories 614 | Total Fat 43.9g 56% | Total Carbohydrate 5.1g 2% | Dietary Fiber 0.2g 1% | Protein 50.9g

— Cheddar Quiche —

Prep: 8 Minutes | Cook Time: 12 Minutes | Makes: 2 Servings

Ingredients:

- 6 eggs, organic
- 1-¼ cup heavy cream
- Salt and black pepper, to taste
- 6 broccoli florets, chopped
- ½ cup cheddar cheese, shredded

Directions:

1. Whisk eggs in a large bowl. Then add heavy cream and whisk it well. Season the mixture with salt and black pepper. Add chopped broccoli florets and cheddar cheese. Now oil greases a quiche dish and pours this mixture into it.
2. Add it into the air fryer basket and adjust the basket inside the unit. Close the unit. Set the time to 12 minutes at 325 ° F (160°C). Once done, serve hot.

Per serving:

Calories 510 | Total Fat 44.7g 57%| Total Carbohydrate 3.1g 1% | Dietary Fiber 0g 0% | Protein 24.9g

— Simple Breakfast Casserole —

Prep: 15 Minutes | Cook Time: 16 Minutes | Makes: 4 Servings

Ingredients:

- 1 pound (450gr) ground sausage
- ½ cup white onion, diced
- 1 green bell pepper, diced
- 1 teaspoon olive oil for greasing
- ½ cup shredded Colby jack cheese
- 8-9 organic eggs, beaten
- 1 teaspoon fennel Seed
- ½ teaspoon garlic Salt

Directions:

1. Preheat the air fryer for 4 minutes at 400 ° F (205°C). Meanwhile, take a large skillet and put sausage in it, along with onion and bell pepper. Cook it for 4 minutes until veggies get slightly soft.
2. Take an air fryer pan and grease it with olive oil. Transfer the sausage mixture to the greased pan. Now at this stage, top it with Colby cheese. Take a separate bowl and whisk eggs in it. Season the eggs with fennel seeds and garlic salt.
3. Then transfer the eggs on top of the cheese and sausage mix. Add the air fryer pan inside and let it air fry for 16 minutes at 330 ° F (165°C). Once done, serve by removing it from the air fryer. Enjoy.

Per serving:

Calories 593 | Total Fat 46.7g 60% | Total Carbohydrate 5.3g 2% | Dietary Fiber 0.9g 3% | Protein 36.7g

— Kale Pancakes —

Prep: 15 Minutes | Cook Time: 15 Minutes | Makes: 2 Servings

Ingredients:

- 2 cups kale leaves, washed
- 1 cup almond flour
- 2.5 cups almond milk
- 1 teaspoon of baking soda
- Pinch of salt
- 1 teaspoon of dried mixed herbs
- ½ teaspoon of garlic powder
- Olive oil spray, as needed

Directions:

1. First, wash the kale leaves and remove the stems. Chop the kale and add it to a high-speed blender with all the listed ingredients. It will be a smooth batter for pancakes at the end. Let it rest for 8 minutes. Grease a cake pan with oil spray. Pour this batter into the cake pan to form a pancake shape.
2. Put a generous amount and fill it appropriately, as we are working in batches.
3. For an air fryer oven, you can use multiple cake pans and air fry 3-4 pancakes at a time. Now add the cake pan to the air fryer.
4. Air fry the pancake for 3-4 minutes (this time depends on its thickness as well) at 350 ° F (180°C). Take it out and air fry the remaining batter, following the same steps. Continue until you have used all the pancake batter. Serve the pancakes with the topping of butter, and enjoy.

Per serving:

Calories 675 | Total Fat 64.2g 82% | Total Carbohydrate 24g 9% | Dietary Fiber 8g 29% | Protein 10.7g

— Breakfast Bacon —

Prep: 15 Minutes | Cook Time: 6-8 Minutes | Makes: 4 Servings

Ingredients:

- 1 pound (450gr) bacon

Directions:

1. Preheat the air fryer for 4 minutes at 350 ° F (180°C). Take an air fryer basket and line the basket with parchment paper. Layer the bacon slices into the basket in a single layer. Do not overlap.
2. Add a basket to the unit. Close the unit. Turn on the air-fry mode and adjust the time to 6-8 minutes. Adjust the temperature to 400 ° F (205°C). Once the bacon gets crispy, take it out, and serve.

Per serving:

Calories 613 | Total Fat 47.4g 61% | Total Carbohydrate 1.6g 1% | Dietary Fiber 0g 0% | Protein 42g

— Breakfast Bombs —

Prep: 20 Minutes | Cook Time: 8-10 Minutes | Makes: 4Servings

Ingredients:

- 4 hardboiled eggs, chopped
- 4 ounces (115gr) of cream cheese
- 2 tablespoons onion, minced
- 1 pound (450gr) of cooked bacon, crumbled

Directions:

1. Preheat the air fryer for 5 minutes to 350 ° F (180°C). Add hard boil eggs, cream Cheese, and onion, and make small balls with your hands. Now roll these balls into bacon crumble. Once coated, mist it with oil spray.
2. Add it to an air fryer basket lined with parchment paper. Set the temperate to 350 ° F (180°C). Set time to 8-10 minutes. Till now, the bacon should be crispy. Take out and serve.

Per serving:

Calories 777 | Total Fat 61.7g 79% | Total Carbohydrate 3.2g 1% | Dietary Fiber 0.1g 0% | Protein 49.7g

— Easy Pancakes —

Prep:15 Minutes | Cook Time: 8 -16 Minutes | Makes: 4 Servings

Ingredients:

- 1 cup of almond flour
- 2 tablespoons coconut flour
- 1 teaspoon baking soda
- 4 large eggs
- 4 tablespoons butter, melted
- ½ cup of soy milk
- 1 teaspoon vanilla extract
- 2 tablespoons water, Pinch of salt

Topping Ingredients:

- 1 cup blueberries
- ½ cup peanut butter

Directions:

1. Preheat the air fryer for 6 minutes at 320 ° F (160°C). Add almond flour, coconut flour, baking soda, and salt, and mix it well. Whisk eggs in a separate bowl and melted butter, soymilk, and vanilla extract. Then add water, whisk it and add it to the flour mixture. Grease a cake pan and pour this batter into it
2. Add the cake pan to the air fryer basket, work in batches, and air fry for 5-8 minutes at 350 ° F(180°C). Work the remaining batter by repeating the steps.
3. Once all the pancakes are done, serve with toppings.

Per serving:

Calories 518| Total Fat 39.4 g 61% | Total Carbohydrate 25 g 8% | Dietary Fiber 10g 38% | Protein 2g

— Cottage Cheese Pancakes —

Prep: 15 Minutes | Cook Time: 6-12 Minutes | Makes: 1 Serving

Ingredients:

- 4 large eggs
- 1 teaspoon of ground Psyllium husk powder
- 1 cup of cottage cheese
- Pinch of salt
- Oil spray for greasing

Topping:

- 2 tablespoons of butter
- 1 cup blueberries

Directions:

1. Whisk eggs in a bowl. Then add Psyllium husk, cottage cheese, and salt. Mix it well again. Sit it for a while until it gets slightly thick.
2. Now pour this batter into the oil-greased basket of the air fryer according to capacity. Add the basket to the unit and air fry it for 6-8 minutes at 360 ° F (180°C) . Once done, serve with a dollop of butter.

Per serving:

Calories 772 | Total Fat 48.3g 62% | Total Carbohydrate 28.6g 10% | Dietary Fiber 4.2g 15% | Protein 57.1g

— Bacon Egg Muffins —

Prep: 15 Minutes | Cook Time: 15 Minutes | Makes: 4 Servings

Ingredients:

- 8 eggs
- 1/3 cup heavy cream
- ½ teaspoon dry mustard powder
- Salt and black pepper to taste
- 4 ounces (115gr) of cheddar cheese shredded
- 8 slices bacon cooked and crumbled
- 2 green onions
- 2 tablespoons fresh parsley or fresh herbs

Directions:

1. Preheat the air fryer to 300 ° F (150°C). Whisk eggs in a large bowl. Add heavy cream, dry mustard, salt, and black pepper to the eggs and whisk it well. Take 8 ramekins and grease them with oil spray.
2. Divide the egg mixture amongst ramekins. Divide the cheese, bacon, and onions over the eggs, and top it with parsley.
3. Air fry it for 15 minutes at 300 ° F (150°C). Once done, take it out and serve.

Per serving:

Calories 448 | Total Fat 36.7g 47% | Total Carbohydrate 2.2g 1% | Dietary Fiber 0.3g 1% | Protein 29.2g

Roasted Red Pepper and Ricotta Frittata

Prep: 12 Minutes | Cook Time: 12 Minutes | Makes: 4 Servings

Ingredients:

- 8 large eggs
- ¼ cup heavy whipping cream
- 1 tablespoon olive oil
- 3 cups raw spinach
- 4 pieces of roasted red peppers chopped
- ½ cup of ricotta cheese

Directions:

1. The first step is to preheat the air fryer for 5 minutes to 350 ° F (180°C). Meanwhile, take a bowl and whisk the egg in it. Then add heavy cream and stir well. Now take a skillet and heat the oil in it. Add spinach and roasted peppers. Let it cook until the spinach wilted. Let it get cool by adding it to a separate plate.
2. Now add the egg mixture to an oil-greased cake pan. Top it with spinach mixture and ricotta cheese.
3. Add it to the air fryer basket. Add the basket to the unit and close the unit. Air fry it at 350° F (180°C) for 10-12 minutes. Serve.

Per serving:

Calories 247 | Total Fat 18.8g 24% | Total Carbohydrate 3.4g 1% | Dietary Fiber 0.5g 2% | Protein 16.9g

— No Grain Bread —

Prep: 12 Minutes | Cook Time: 15 Minutes | Makes: 2 Servings

Ingredients:

- 4 tablespoons Psyllium husk powder
- ½ cup almond flour
- 1 teaspoon of baking soda
- 8 tablespoons cottage cheese
- 8 tablespoons egg white
- Oil spray for greasing, Pinch of salt

Directions:

1. Take a bowl and add Psyllium, almond flour, salt, and cottage cheese. Then whisk egg whites in a separate bowl and add them to the flour mixture. Shape mixture into buns. Mist buns with oil spray. Add buns to an air fryer basket lined with parchment paper
2. Add the basket to the air fryer. Close the air fryer. Air fry it at 320 ° F 160°C) for 15 minutes, flipping halfway through. Remove it from the air fryer, let it sit for a few minutes, and then serve.

Per serving:

Calories 288 | Total Fat 14.8g 19% | Total Carbohydrate 18.5g 7% | Dietary Fiber 12g 43% | Protein 20.4g

Hard Boiled Eggs for Breakfast

Prep: 10 Minutes | Cook Time: 16-18 Minutes | Makes: 2Servings

Ingredients:

- 4 large eggs

Directions:

1. Preheat the air fryer to 300 ° F (150°C) for 2 minutes. Add the eggs to the basket of the air fryer. Add the basket to the unit and close the air fryer.
2. Air fry it at 280 ° F (140°C) for 16-18 minutes. Once done, add into a cold water bowl to stop the cooking process. Peel the eggs and serve with them.

Per serving:

Calories 143 | Total Fat 9.9g 13% | Total Carbohydrate 0.8g 0% | Dietary Fiber 0g 0% | Protein 12.6g

Fluffy Chocolate Chip Pancakes

Prep: 12 Minutes | Cook Time: 8-16 Minutes | Makes: 3 Servings

Ingredients:

- 2 tablespoons coconut flour
- 1 cup almond flour
- 1 tablespoon Psyllium husk
- 1 teaspoon baking soda
- 5 eggs
- 6 tablespoons butter, melted
- 8 drops flavored liquid stevia
- ¼ cup dark chocolate chips, divided
- Olive oil spray for greasing

Side Serving:

- 4 tablespoons of butter

Directions:

1. Take a bowl and add coconut flour, almond flour, Psyllium, and baking soda. Then, whisk eggs in a separate bowl, and add melted butter and stevia. Combine both bowl mixtures.
2. Now pour this batter into the oil-greased basket of the air fryer according to capacity. Top it with some chocolate chips. Work in batches here.
3. Add the basket to the unit and air fry it for 6-8 minutes at 350 ° F (180°C). Do not flip the pancakes.
4. Work the remaining batter by repeating the steps. Once all the pancakes are done, serve with a dollop of butter.

Per serving:

Calories 535 | Total Fat 45.1g 58% | Total Carbohydrate 23.2g 8% | Dietary Fiber 15.7g 56% | Protein 14.2g

— Chicken, Bell Peppers Quiche —

Prep: 15 Minutes | Cook Time: 16 Minutes | Makes: 2 Servings

Ingredients:

- 4 organic eggs
- Salt and black pepper, to taste
- 1/3 cup Parmesan cheese, shredded
- 4 tablespoons green bell pepper, chopped
- Oil spray for greasing
- 1 cup chicken, cooked and crumbled

Directions:

1. Preheat the air fryer for 4 minutes at 350 ° F (180°C). Crack and whisk the eggs in a bowl and season the eggs with salt and black pepper. Then add cheese and chopped bell peppers and mix them well
2. Grease 4 ramekins with oil spray. Divide the egg mixture among the ramekins. Top with crumbles of chicken. Add it to air fryer baskets. Add the basket to the unit and closet the air fryer. Air fry it for 12-16 minutes at 350 ° F (180°C). Once cooked, serve it hot and enjoy.

Per serving:

Calories 359 | Total Fat 14.9g 19% | Total Carbohydrate 19.1g 7% | Dietary Fiber 3.2g 11% | Protein 38.2g

— Easy Breakfast Sausage —

Prep: 10 Minutes | Cook Time: 10 Minutes | Makes: 1 Serving

Ingredients:

- 1 pound (450gr) pork, grounded
- Salt and black pepper, to taste
- ½ teaspoon fennel seeds, crushed slightly
- ½ teaspoon garlic powder
- ½ teaspoon onion powder
- 1/8 teaspoon thyme leaves
- 1/8 teaspoon cayenne pepper
- Oil spray for greasing

Directions:

1. Add ground pork and remaining listed seasoning in a large bowl, mix well and let it rest inside the refrigerator for 2 hours. Afterward, take it out and divide the mixture into patties. Mist the patties with oil spray.
2. Line an air fryer basket with parchment paper. Layer the patties onto the air fryer basket. Add the basket to the unit. Select the air fry mode of the air fryer.
3. Adjust the time to 10 minutes and the temperature to 400 ° F (205°C). Once done, serve.

Per serving:

Calories 667 | Total Fat 16.7g 21% | Total Carbohydrate 2.8g 1% | Dietary Fiber 0.8g 3% | Protein 119.3g

Walnut and Almond Meal Muffins

Prep: 15 Minutes | Cook Time: 10 Minutes | Makes: 2 Servings

Ingredients:

- 1-¼ cup almond flour
- 1 teaspoon baking powder
- ¼ cup stevia
- 2 organic eggs
- 1/3 cup almond milk
- 2 tablespoons butter
- 1 teaspoon of orange zest
- ¼ cup orange juice
- ½ cup walnuts, chopped. Pinch of salt

Directions:

1. Preheat the air fryer to 300 ° F (150°C) for 5 minutes. Incorporate almond flour, baking powder, salt, and stevia. Take a separate bowl and crack eggs in it.
2. Then whisk the eggs and add almond milk, butter, orange zest, and orange juice. Fold in the walnuts at the end. Divide this muffin batter among ramekins that are lined with muffin cups.
3. Air fry the muffins in batches inside the basket for 10 minutes at 350 ° F (180°C). Once it's done, serve and enjoy.

Per serving:

Calories 551 | Total Fat 50.6g 65% | Total Carbohydrate 13.3g 5% | Dietary Fiber 4.7g 17% | Protein 17.3g

— Broccoli Omelet —

Prep: 22 Minutes | Cook Time: 12 Minutes | Makes: 3 Servings

Ingredients:

- 6 eggs, beaten
- 1 cup broccoli florets steamed
- 2 medium button mushrooms, sliced
- 1/3 cup shredded cheese Mexican Blend
- 1 tablespoon coconut milk
- Salt and black pepper, to taste
- Oil spray for greasing

Directions:

1. Grease a small cake pan with oil spray. Whisk eggs in a bowl. Then add the entire list one by one and keep stirring. Pour this batter into greased cake pan.
2. Add the cake pan to the air fryer and cook for 10-12 minutes at 320 ° F (160°C). The eggs should get firm now.

Per serving:

Calories 149 | Total Fat 10.9g 14% | Total Carbohydrate 1.1g 0% | Dietary Fiber 0.1g 0% | Protein 11.9g

Egg, Cheese, Bacon, and Ham Cups

Prep: 15 Minutes | Cook Time: 10 Minutes | Makes: 2 Servings

Ingredients:

- 4 eggs, whisked
- 2 tablespoons almond milk
- 4 ham slices, chopped
- ½ cup Mexican cheese, grated
- 1 green onion, diced
- Salt and pepper, to taste

Directions:

1. Preheat the air fryer to 355 ° F (180°C) for a few minutes. Meanwhile, take a muffin tin or 4 ramekins and line them with muffin paper. Whisk eggs in a bowl and pour in the almond milk. Then whisk again and add Ham, Cheese, onions, salt, and black pepper. Equally, pour this amongst ramekins and add the ramekins to the air fryer basket.
2. Add the basket to the unit. Close the unit. Air fry it for 10 minutes at 356 ° F (185°C). Once done, serve.

Per serving:

Calories 277 | Total Fat 22.1g 28% | Total Carbohydrate 3.6g 1% | Dietary Fiber 0.6g 2%| Protein 19.4g

Prosciutto and Spinach Egg Cups

Prep: 15 Minutes | Cook Time 12 Minutes | Makes: 2 Servings

Ingredients:

- Oil spray for greasing
- 4 slices of prosciuttos
- ¼ cup of spinach leaves
- 4 eggs, whisked
- 4 tablespoons of cheddar cheese
- Salt and black pepper, to taste
- 2 teaspoons of chives, chopped

Directions:

1. Take four ramekins and mist them with oil spray from the bottom. Now layer the bottom with equal proportions of the prosciutto. Then top it with a generous amount of spinach and pour the whisked eggs on top of each ramekin. Top it with cheddar cheese, salt, and pepper.
2. Palace it inside an air fryer basket. Add a basket to the unit. Close the unit. Air fry it at 350 ° F (180°C) for 10-12 minutes. Serve with a topping of chives.

Per serving:

Calories 307 | Total Fat 19.7g 25% | Total Carbohydrate 1.1g 0% | Dietary Fiber 0.1g 0% | Protein 30.8g

Eggs and Cheese Muffin

Prep: 15 Minutes | Cook Time: 15 Minutes | Makes: 4 Servings

Ingredients:

- 8 eggs
- ½ cup of grated cheddar Cheese
- Salt and pepper according to taste

Directions:

1. Take 4 ramekins, grease them with oil spray, and set them aside for further use. Whisk eggs in a bowl and add salt and black pepper. Add the cheddar cheese to the egg mixture and whisk. Equally, divide this mixture among the ramekins
2. Add the ramekins to the air fryer basket. Add the basket to the air fryer. Close the unit. Air fry it for 15 minutes at 350 ° F (180°C). Work in batches according to the capacity of the air fryer basket.

Per serving:

Calories 242 | Total Fat 15.3g 20%| Total Carbohydrate 1.7g 1% | Dietary Fiber 0g 0% | Protein 25.1g

Banana and Chocolate Chip Muffins

Prep: 15 Minutes | Cook Time: 12 Minutes | Makes: 2 Servings

Ingredients:

- Salt, pinch
- 1.5 cups almond flour
- ½ teaspoon of baking powder
- 2 eggs, whisked
- 4 tablespoons of coconut milk
- 2 tablespoons butter, melted
- 1 cup mashed bananas
- 4 tablespoons of chocolate chip

Directions:

1. The first step is to preheat the air fryer for 5 minutes to 350 ° F (180°C). Combine salt, almond flour, and baking powder in a bowl. In a separate bowl, whisk eggs and add coconut milk and butter.
2. Now add the mashed bananas and chocolate chips. Now incorporate dry ingredients with wet ingredients. Line the ramekins with muffin paper. Divide this batter amongst ramekins.
3. Add the ramekins inside the basket of the air fryer. Air fry for 10-12 minutes at 400 ° F (205°C). Once it's done, serve and enjoy.

Per serving:

Calories 249| Total Fat 18.1g 23% | Total Carbohydrate 17.6g 6% | Dietary Fiber 2.4g 9% | Protein 5.9g

Egg Bites with Deli Turkey and Chives

Prep: 10 Minutes | Cook Time: 15 Minutes | Makes: 2 Servings

Ingredients:

- 10 large eggs
- Salt and black pepper, to taste
- ½ cup almond milk
- 6 ounces (170gr) deli turkey, finely chopped
- 2 teaspoons dried chives, finely chopped

Directions:

1. Take an air fryer-proof dish that fits inside the basket of an air fryer. Line the dish with parchment paper and set it aside. Crack eggs in a large bowl and whisk with salt and black pepper. Then add almond milk and whisk it well using an immersion blender.
2. Now add deli turkey and chives and stir it well. Pour this egg mixture into the baking dish.
3. Add it to the basket and place it inside the unit. Close the unit and air fry the egg for 15 minutes at 350°F (180°C). Once the egg gets firm, take it out and into squares and serve.

Per serving:

Calories 591 |Total Fat 41.7g 53% | Total Carbohydrate 11.9g 4% | Dietary Fiber 1.7g 6% | Protein 44.3g

Breakfast Frittata

Prep: 15 Minutes | Cook Time: 12 Minutes | Makes: 2 Servings

Ingredients:

- 4 eggs
- 4 tablespoons of whipping cream
- 1/3 cup of baby spinach
- 6 tablespoons of feta cheese
- ¼cup of cherry tomatoes
- 2 tablespoons of thinly sliced onions
- ½ teaspoons of dried oregano
- Salt and pepper according to taste

Directions:

1. Take a cake pan that fits inside the air fryer basket. Grease the cake pan with oil spray. Whisk the cream and egg in a small bowl to incorporate well.
2. Next, add spinach, feta cheese, tomatoes, onions, oregano, salt, and pepper. Whisk it well. Pour this into a cake pan and cover the pan with aluminum foil
3. Add it to the air fryer basket. Add the basket to the unit. Close the unit. Air fry it for 12 minutes at 350°F (180°C). Once it's done, serve.

Per serving:

Calories 298 | Total Fat 24.1g 31% | Total Carbohydrate 5g 2% | Dietary Fiber 0.8g 3% | Protein 16.2g

Zucchini Egg Cups

Prep: 15 Minutes | Cook Time: 12-15 Minutes | Makes: 4 Servings

Ingredients:

- Oil spray for greasing
- 6-8 eggs
- 1 teaspoon smoked paprika
- Salt and black pepper, to taste
- 1 teaspoon baking powder
- 1 medium zucchini, chopped
- 4 teaspoons of tomato, chopped
- 1 cup fresh spinach, chopped

Directions:

1. Preheat the air fryer for 4 minutes to 350 ° F (180°C). Meanwhile, take a muffin tin that fits inside the backset of the air fryer. Grease the muffin tin with oil spray and set it aside for further use.
2. Crack the eggs in a large bowl and beat until fluffy. Season the egg with smoked paprika, salt, pepper, and baking powder. Drain the zucchini to remove the water, and add it to the egg mixture. Add the tomato and spinach and stir well.
3. Fill the muffin tin with this mixture and add it to the air fryer. Air fry for 12 minutes at 350 ° F (180°C). Once done, take it out and serve the cups.

Per serving:

Calories 119 | Total Fat 7g 9% | Total Carbohydrate 5.7g 2% | Dietary Fiber 1.7g 6% | Protein 9.7g

Crab and Shrimp Omelet

Prep: 20 Minutes | Cook Time: 8-10 Minutes | Makes: 1-2 Servings

Ingredients:

- Oil spray for greasing
- 3 large eggs
- Salt and black pepper, to taste
- 2 ounces(60gr) of raw shrimp, peeled and deveined
- 1.5 ounces (40gr) of lump crabmeat
- 1 slice cheese, your choice

Directions:

1. Take a cake pan and mist it with oil spray. Whisk eggs in a bowl and add salt and pepper. Now whisk it well again.
2. Add the cake pan to the air fryer and cook for 4 minutes at 350 ° F(180°C).
3. Once 4 minutes pass, take the cake, pan put, and top it with shrimp and crabmeat pieces, along with cheese. Air fry it for 4 minutes more. Then serve.

Per serving:

Calories 222 | Total Fat 13.2g 17% | Total Carbohydrate 1.2g 0% | Dietary Fiber 0g 0% | Protein 23.7g

Mushroom and Ground Beef Stuffed Omelet

Prep: 15 Minutes | Cook Time: 25-30 Minutes | Makes: 2-3 Servings

Ingredients for Mushroom Filling:

- 2 tablespoons extra virgin olive oil
- 8 ounces (230gr) of brown button mushrooms
- 1 tablespoon coconut aminos
- ½ tablespoon balsamic vinegar
- 1 tablespoon stevia
- 2 tablespoons butter
- ½ sprig of thyme, chopped
- Salt and pepper, to taste

Ingredients for Ground Beef filling:

- 1 tablespoon olive oil
- 1 cup of ground beef
- 1 teaspoon Thai curry paste
- Salt and black pepper to taste

Basic Omelets:

- 6 eggs
- Salt, to taste
- 2 teaspoons unsalted butter

Toppings:

- 1/3 cup cheddar cheese or parmesan cheese, grated

Directions:

1. First, prepare the Mushroom Filling. For that, heat the oil in a skillet and add mushrooms. Then add coconut aminos, vinegar, and stevia. Cook it for 5 minutes at low flame. Now add the butter. Mix the ingredients well and add thyme. Sauté it for 4 minutes. Season it with salt and black pepper and set aside.
2. Now prepare the beef filling. For that, heat 1 tablespoon of oil in a pan and cook ground beef with Thai curry paste, salt, and pepper. Cook it for 7 minutes at 400 ° F (205°C).
3. Now prepare an omelet. Take a cake pan that fits inside the basket of the air fryer. Now whisk eggs in a bowl, season it with salt, and add the butter.
4. Transfer the egg to the cake pan and add the cake pan to the air fryer basket. Add the basket to the unit. Air fry the eggs at 350 ° F (180°C) for 6 minutes.
5. Take it out and transfer it to the plate. Now top it with mushroom and beef fillings. Sprinkle cheese on top. Again place it back into the air fryer. Air fry for 3 more minutes. Till now, the omelet would be set. Take out and serve.

Per serving:

Calories 471 | Total Fat 39.2g 50% | Total Carbohydrate 4.5g 2% | Dietary Fiber 0.5g 2% | Protein 26.4g

— Mug Muffins —

Prep: 10 Minutes | Cook Time: 8 Minutes | Makes: 1 Serving

Ingredients:

- Oil spray for greasing
- 4 teaspoons of coconut flour
- ½ teaspoon baking soda
- Salt, pinch
- 2 eggs
- 4 tablespoons feta cheese, shredded cheddar cheese
- 2 teaspoons basil, roughly chopped

Directions:

1. Preheat the air fryer for 4 minutes to 350 ° F (180°C). Meanwhile, take the large coffee mug and grease it with oil spray. Then, add coconut flour, baking soda, and a pinch of salt and whisk the egg.
2. Next, add the feta cheese and basil. Mix it well, and then scoop this batter into a mug
3. Add it to the air fryer basket. Add the basket to the unit. Air fry it at 350 ° F (180°C) for 6-8 minutes. Once done, take out and serve.

Per serving:

Calories 118 | Total Fat 6.3g 8% | Total Carbohydrate 8.6g 3% | Dietary Fiber 5g 18% | Protein 6.1g

— Rainbow Omelet —

Prep: 20 Minutes | Cook Time: 8-10 Minutes | Makes: 1-2 Servings

Ingredients:

- Oil spray for greasing and misting
- 4 eggs, whisked
- ½ small onion, diced
- ¼ small red bell pepper, diced
- ¼ small green bell pepper, diced
- ¼ small yellow bell pepper, diced
- ½ cup ham, diced
- ¼ cup cheddar cheese, shredded
- Salt and black pepper to taste

Directions:

1. Take a cake pan and mist it with oil spray. Whisk eggs in a bowl and add onions, listed bell peppers, ham, and cheese. Then season it with salt and black pepper. Whisk all the ingredients well. Pour this into the cake pan.
2. Add the cake pan to the air fryer basket. Add the basket to the unit. Air fry it for 8-10 minutes at 350°F (180°C). Then serve.

Per serving:

Calories 258 | Total Fat 16.7g 21% | Total Carbohydrate 6.4g 2% | Dietary Fiber 1.5g 5% | Protein 20.8g

Sour Cream and Onion Omelet

Prep: 22 Minutes | Cook Time: 10-12 Minutes | Makes: 2 Servings

Ingredients:
- 4 large eggs
- 2 ounces (60gr) cheese, shredded
- 1 ounce (30gr) red onion, finely diced
- 2 tablespoons sour cream, room temperature
- Salt and ground black pepper, to taste
- 2 teaspoons butter

Directions:
1. Preheat the air fryer for 4 minutes to 400 ° F (205°C). Whisk eggs in a bowl. Then add cheese, onion, sour cream, salt, and pepper. Grease a cake pan with butter and pour the mixture inside it.
2. Add it to the air fryer basket. Add a basket to the unit. Air fry at 350 ° F (180°C) for 10-12 minutes until the egg gets firm with your preferred doneness. Serve.

Per serving:

Calories 322 | Total Fat 25.7g 33% | Total Carbohydrate 3g 1% | Dietary Fiber 0.3g 1% | Protein 20.2g

Blueberry Muffins

Prep: 15 Minutes | Cook Time: 8-10 Minutes | Makes 4 Servings

Ingredients:
- 2.5 cups of almond flour
- ½ cup monk fruit blend
- 1.5 teaspoons baking soda
- 1/3 cup butter, melted
- 1/3 cup coconut milk
- 3 large organic eggs, Sea salt, pinch
- ½ teaspoon vanilla extract
- 3/4 cup blueberries, fresh and washed

Directions:
1. Preheat the air fryer for 4 minutes to 350 ° F (180°C). Take ramekins and line them ramekins with muffin paper. Mix well in a bowl and combine almond flour, monk fruit blend, baking soda, and sea salt.
2. In a separate bowl, whisk butter and coconut milk. Crack eggs into this mixture. Whisk and add it to the flour mixture. Incorporate all the ingredients well.
3. Add vanilla extract, mix the blueberries, and dump the dollops into ramekins. Add it to the basket and bake for about 8-10 minutes at 350 ° F (180°C). Once done, serve.

Per serving:

Calories 252 | Total Fat 23.9g 31% | Total Carbohydrate 5.4g 2% | Dietary Fiber 1.1g 4% | Protein 5.6g

Salmon Breakfast Egg Bites

Prep: 20 Minutes | Cook Time: 12-15 Minutes | Makes: 5 Servings

Ingredients:
- 10 large eggs
- Salt and black pepper, to taste
- 1 cup coconut milk
- 3 ounces (85gr) of smoked salmon, cut into strips
- 2 teaspoons fresh dill, chopped

Directions:
1. Preheat the air fryer for 4 minutes at 350 ° F (180°C). Meanwhile, take a heatproof baking dish. Line the dish with parchment paper and set it aside.
2. Crack eggs in a large bowl and whisk with salt and black pepper using an immersion blender. Then add coconut milk and whisk it well. Pour this egg mixture into the baking dish, and then top it with smoked salmon and dill.
3. Add it to the air fryer basket of the unit. Close the team, and air fry the egg for 12-15 minutes at 350 ° F (180°C). Once the egg gets firm, take it out and into squares and serve.

Per serving:

Calories 274 | Total Fat 22.1g 28% | Total Carbohydrate 3.7g 1% | Dietary Fiber 1.1g 4% | Protein 16.9g

Baked Egg Cups with Bacon and Cheese

Prep: 12 Minutes | Cook Time: 6 Minutes | Makes: 1 Serving

Ingredients:
- 2 eggs
- 2 teaspoons almond milk
- 2 teaspoons cheddar cheese, grated
- Salt and pepper, according to taste
- 4 teaspoons of bacon bits
- Oil spray for greasing

Directions:
1. Grease the 2 ramekins with oil spray. Set aside for further use. Take a bowl and crack eggs in it for whisking. Then add almond milk and whisk again.
2. Now add cheese, salt, and black pepper. Mix everything well. Now add bacon bits and stir so it combines. Pour this egg batter into ramekins.
3. Add the ramekin to the air fryer basket. Add a basket to the unit. Close the unit. Air fry it at 370 ° F (190°C) for 6 minutes. Once done, serve.

Per serving:

Calories 146 | Total Fat 11.3g 14% | Total Carbohydrate 0.6g 0% | Dietary Fiber 0.1g 0% | Protein 10.2g

Omelet with Deli Ham and Cheese

Prep: 12 Minutes | Cook Time: 8-12 Minutes | Makes: 1-2 Servings

Ingredients:

- 3 large organic eggs
- Salt and pepper, to taste
- ¼ cup of coriander, roughly chopped
- 3 ounces (85gr) deli ham roughly chopped
- 4 tablespoons cheddar cheese, shredded
- 1 teaspoon butter
- ¼ teaspoon hot sauce

Directions:

1. Whisk eggs in a bowl, and then season them with salt and pepper. Whisk it and add coriander, Ham, and Cheese. Grease a cake pan with butter from the bottom. Pour this egg mixture into the cake pan.
2. Add the cake pan to the air fryer basket. Add the basket to the unit. Close the door. Set the time to 350 ° F (180°C) for 8-12 minutes.
3. Once the egg gets firm, take it out and serve the delicious omelet with hot sauce.

Per serving:

Calories 227 | Total Fat 15.6g 20% | Total Carbohydrate 0.9g 0% | Dietary Fiber 0.1g 0% | Protein 19.9g

Oatmeal without Oats

Prep: 12 Minutes | Cook Time: 8-12 Minutes | Makes: 2 Servings

Ingredients:

- Oil spray for greasing
- 1 scoop of chocolate protein powder
- 4 tablespoons almond flour
- 4 tablespoons unsweetened shredded coconut
- 1 tablespoon ground flax seed
- ½ cup of unsweetened coconut milk

Optional Topping:

- 2 tablespoons Shredded Coconut
- 1/3 cup of blueberries
- 2 tablespoons Cacao Nibs
- 2 tablespoons Pumpkin Seeds

Directions:

1. Grease a cake pan with oil spray. Add all the listed ingredients, excluding toppings, into a round small cake pan. Mix it and add it to the air fryer basket.
2. Add the basket to the unit and close the unit. Air fry it at 350 ° F (180°C) for 8-12 minutes.
3. Take it from the air fryer and serve it with the listed toppings.

Per serving:

Calories 615 | Total Fat 50.6g 65% | Total Carbohydrate 28.1g 10% | Dietary Fiber 12.9g 46% | Protein 16.8g

Green Chili Eggs

Prep: 14 Minutes | Cook Time: 8 Minutes | Makes: 3 Servings

Ingredients:

- 6 eggs, whisked
- ½ cup half and half
- 2 small green chilies, chopped
- 2 teaspoons of green onions, chopped
- Salt, to taste
- ¼ teaspoon ground cumin
- ¼ cup cheddar cheese

Directions:

1. Take a bowl and crack eggs in it. Then add half and half green chilies, green onions, salt, cumin, and cheddar cheese. Whisk it well.
2. Pour this into the cake pan.
3. Add the cake pan to the air fryer basket. Add the basket to the unit. Air fry it for 8-10 minutes at 350°F (180°C). Then serve.

Per serving:

Calories 228 | Total Fat 16.6g 21% | Total Carbohydrate 5.2g 2% | Dietary Fiber 0.7g 2% | Protein 15.1g

Peanut Butter Porridge

Prep: 15 Minutes | Cook Time: 8-10 Minutes | Makes: 4 Servings

Ingredients:

- 2 tablespoons flaxseed meal, golden
- 2 tablespoons coconut flour
- 2 tablespoons chia seeds
- ½ cup unsweetened almond milk
- 2 tablespoons heavy cream
- 2-3 tablespoons stevia
- 1 teaspoon vanilla essence

Toppings:

- 4 pecans, chopped
- 2 tablespoons of peanut butter

Directions:

1. Take a heatproof air fryer-safe bowl and add all the dry ingredients. Then add to the dry ingredients listed amount of almond milk, heavy cream, stevia, and vanilla essence. Mix it and add it to the bowl.
2. Place bowl into air fryer basket. Add a basket to the unit. Close the unit. Air fry at 375 ° F (190°C) for 8-10 minutes. It should be thickened till now.
3. Top it with chopped pecans and a dollop of peanut butter.

Per serving:

Calories 232 | Total Fat 20.6g 26% | Total Carbohydrate 8.7g 3% | Dietary Fiber 6.1g 22% | Protein 5.9g

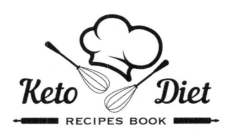

Chapter

5

Simple Recipes

—= Lamb Meatballs =—

Prep: 25 Minutes | Cook Time: 15 Minutes | Makes: 2 Servings

Ingredients:
- 1 pound (450gr) ground lamb meat
- 1 egg
- ½ cup almond flour
- ¼ cup parmesan cheese
- 1 teaspoon cumin, grounded
- 4 teaspoons onions, grounded
- 4 tablespoons parsley
- Salt and black pepper, to taste
- 1 cup mozzarella cheese, cubed
- oil spray for greasing

Directions:
1. Add lamb meat, egg, almond flour, parmesan cheese, cumin, onion, parsley, salt, and black pepper. Mix it well. Make round meatballs and add one cube of cheese into the center, sealing the sides. Repeat the steps until all the remaining meatballs are ready. Mist the meatballs with oil spray.
2. Add it to the air fryer basket and add the basket to the unit. Air fry it for 15 minutes at 400 ° F (205°C). Once it's done, serve.

Per serving:

Calories 639 | Total Fat 35g 45% | Total Carbohydrate 25g 9% | Dietary Fiber 5.5g 20% | Protein 52.9g

—= Lemon Ricotta Cake =—

Prep: 15 Minutes | Cook Time: 20 Minutes| Makes: 4 Servings

Ingredients:
- 2 egg whites
- 2 egg yolks
- 1 teaspoon salt
- ¾ cup stevia
- 1-1/3 cup butter (melted)
- 1 cup almond flour
- 1 tablespoon baking soda
- 1 cup ricotta cheese
- 1 lemon, zest only

Directions:
1. Take a bowl and whisk egg whites in it. Once a stiff peak forms on to,p set it aside. Take a separate bowl and add egg yolks with salt, stevia, butter, almond flour, baking soda, cheese, and lemon zest. Whisk all these ingredients very well. Now add egg whites to this mixture.
2. Grease a cake pan with oil spray. Pour this batter into the cake pan.
3. Put the cake pan inside the air fryer basket. Add the basket to the unit. Bake it for 20 minutes at 320 ° F (160°C).Make sure to check the cake during the cooking cycle. Once done, serve and enjoy.

Per serving:

Calories 329 |Total Fat 24g 31% | Total Carbohydrate 11.1g 4% | Dietary Fiber 3.8g 13% | Protein 17.7g

— Roasted Purple Cauliflower —

Prep: 10 Minutes | Cook Time: 12 Minutes | Makes: 4 Servings

Ingredients for Purple Cauliflower

- 1 small head of purple cauliflower cut into florets
- 2 tablespoons avocado oil
- Salt and black pepper, to taste
- 2 pinches of paprika

Directions:

1. Add the cauliflower florets to a large bowl and add avocado oil, salt, pepper, and paprika. Line an air fryer basket with parchment paper.
2. Add the cauliflower florets into the basket. Add the basket to the unit. Close the air fryer. Air fry it for 12 minutes at 400 ° F (205°C).Once done, serve and enjoy.

Per serving:

Calories 13 | Total Fat 1g 1% | Total Carbohydrate 1g 0% | Dietary Fiber 0.7g 2% | Protein 0.4g

— Spicy Veggies with Cheese —

Prep: 20 Minutes | Cook Time: 22 Minutes | Makes: 2 Servings

Ingredients:

- 1 head cauliflower cut into florets
- 2 teaspoons of olive oil
- ¾ cup white onion, thinly sliced
- 3 cloves garlic finely sliced
- 1-½ tablespoons tamari
- 1 tablespoon rice vinegar
- ½ teaspoon stevia
- Salt and black pepper, to taste
- 1 tablespoon Sriracha sauce
- 2 scallions, chopped for garnish
- ½ cup parmesan cheese, grated, Salt, to taste

Directions:

1. Preheat the air fryer for 4 minutes at 400 ° F (205°C). Take an air fryer basket, grease it with oil spray, or line it with parchment paper. Toss cauliflower with salt and olive oil.
2. Add it to the air fryer basket and cook it for 12 minutes at 400 ° F (205°C).
3. Take out the basket, add sliced onion, and air fry it for 8 more minutes.
4. Meanwhile, take a bowl and whisk all the remaining listed ingredients. Toss it over cooked veggies in an air fryer and top with parmesan cheese.
5. Air fry it for 2 more minutes at 400 ° F (205°C) until the cheese melts. Once it has been done, serve.

Per serving:

Calories 326 | Total Fat 16.9g 22% | Total Carbohydrate 23.4g 8% | Dietary Fiber 4.4g 16% | Protein 23g

— Rocket Pancakes —

Prep: 12 Minutes | Cook Time: 6-8 Minutes | Makes: 4 Servings

Ingredients:

- 2 cups of almond flour
- 2 eggs, whisked
- 1 tablespoon baking soda
- 1/3 cup melted butter
- Salt, just a pinch or more
- 1-2 cups water
- 1/4 cup of red peppers, sliced
- 1/4 cup parsley, chopped
- 2 cups arugula, chopped
- 2 ounces (60gr) chopped prosciutto
- Oil spray for greasing

Directions:

1. Mix the almond flour with eggs, baking soda, butter, salt, and water in a large bowl. Mix it well and add red pepper, parsley, arugula, and prosciutto. Make a smooth pancake batter. Now take a cake pan and grease the pan with oil spray.
2. Pour the batter into the pan and add the pan to the basket. Add the basket to the unit. Air fry it at 350 ° F (180°C) for 6-8 minutes, flipping halfway.
3. Work in batches and repeat the step unit all batter is consumed. Serve and enjoy.

Per serving:

Calories 275 | Total Fat 25.6g 33% | Total Carbohydrate 4.5g 2% | Dietary Fiber 1.8g 7% | Protein 9.4g

— Classic Tofu Nuggets —

Prep: 12 Minutes | Cook Time: 12 Minutes | Makes: 2 Servings

Ingredients:

- 1 block of tofu, pressed and drained
- Salt and black pepper, to taste
- 1 teaspoon of smoked paprika
- ¼teaspoon garlic powder
- 1 cup almond flour
- Oil spray for greasing

Directions:

1. Cut the tofu into small cubes. Add salt, pepper, smoked paprika, and garlic powder to a large bowl. Toss the tofu with it. Then dust it with an almond flour coating. Mist it with oil spray.
2. Add it to an air fryer basket lined with parchment paper. Bake the tofu for 12 minutes at 400 ° F (205°C), shaking the basket halfway through. Once it's done, serve.

Per serving:

Calories 115 | Total Fat 9.1g 12% | Total Carbohydrate 4.6g 2% | Dietary Fiber 2.3g 8% | Protein 6.5g

— Zucchini Tots —

Prep: 20 Minutes | Cook Time: 12 Minutes | Makes: 4 Servings

Ingredients:

- 2 medium zucchini
- 1 large egg
- ½ cup grated pecorino
- ½ cup grated parmesan cheese
- ½ cup almond flour
- 1 clove garlic, crushed
- ½ teaspoon of black pepper

Directions:

1. Shred the zucchini and squeeze out excess water. Pat dry it with a paper towel. Add zucchini to a bowl and add eggs, pecorino, parmesan cheese, almonds, flour, garlic, and pepper.
2. Take a cookie scoop to drop tablespoonfuls of mixture onto an air fryer basket lined with parchment paper. Air fry it for 10-12 minutes at 400 ° F (205°C). Once it's done, serve.

Per serving:

Calories 255 | Total Fat 17.2g 22% | Total Carbohydrate 5.6g 2% | Dietary Fiber 1.6g 6% | Protein 19.6g

— Crispy Eggplants —

Prep: 22 Minutes | Cook Time: 15 Minutes | Makes: 4 Servings

Ingredients:

- ¼ teaspoon of red chilies
- ½ teaspoon of coriander
- salt, to taste
- ¼ teaspoon of baking soda
- ¼ teaspoon of dry pomegranate seeds, grated
- 1 cup almond flour
- ½ cup water or more
- 2 cups large eggplants, thin round cuts

Directions:

1. Mix red chilies, coriander, salt, baking soda, dry pomegranate seeds, almond flour, and water to make a smooth paste. It makes a runny batter.
2. Dip the eggplant slices in the batter. Start layering it onto a tray lined with parchment paper. Refrigerate it for 1 hour.
3. Then put the eggplants into an air fryer basket lined with parchment paper. Air fry it for 15 minutes at 400 ° F (205°C), flipping halfway through. Once it's cooked, serve and enjoy.

Per serving:

Calories 55 | Total Fat 3.6g 5% | Total Carbohydrate 5g 2% | Dietary Fiber 2.5g 9% | Protein 2g

— Jicama Cutlets —

Prep: 25 Minutes | Cook Time: 20 Minutes | Makes: 6 Servings

Ingredients:

- 4 jicama, washed and peeled
- 1 cup of mozzarella cheese
- 2 tablespoons of olive oil
- Salt and black pepper, to taste
- ½ teaspoon of oregano
- ½ cup bell pepper, chopped
- 2 eggs, whisked
- ½ cup pork rinds (grated)

Directions:

1. Take a pot and boil water in it. Then add jicama and cook it for 15 minutes. Now add the boiled jicama to a tray. Let it get dry, and pat dry with a paper towel. Add the jicama n a bowl and mash it well. Then mix it with cheese, olive oil, salt, pepper, oregano, and bell pepper. Mix it well.
2. Use your hand to prepare the shapes of cutlets.
3. Whisk eggs in a large bowl. Add pork rinds to a separate bowl. Dip the cutlets in eggs, and then coat them with grated pork rinds.
4. Add it to the air fryer basket and line it with parchment paper. Add the basket to the unit. Air fryer it at 400 ° F (205°C) for 6-8 minutes, flipping halfway through. Once it's done, serve.

Per serving:

Calories 210 | Total Fat 9.7g 12% | Total Carbohydrate 22.6g 8% | Dietary Fiber 12.1g 43% | Protein 9.5g

— Squash Noodles —

Prep: 15 minutes | Cook Time: 8-10 Minutes | Makes: 2 Servings

Ingredients:

- 2 cups squash, spiralized
- Salt and black pepper, to taste
- 2 teaspoons of olive oil
- 1 cup parmesan cheese, grated
- 1 cup peanut sauce, no sugar, and optional

Directions:

1. Put spiralized squash in a colander and add salt. Let it sit for 10 minutes, then squeeze excess water. Now add it to oil greased air fryer basket along with salt, black pepper, and olive oil drizzle.
2. Cook for 10 minutes at 400 ° F (205°C). Once it's cooked, serve it with a topping of parmesan cheese. Enjoy hot with peanut sauce.

Per serving:

Calories 69 | Total Fat 5.6g 7% | Total Carbohydrate 3.9g 1% | Dietary Fiber 1.2g 4% | Protein 2.5g

Artichoke Fries

Prep: 10 Minutes | Cook Time: 18 Minutes | Makes: 2-4 Servings

Ingredients:

- 16 ounces (450gr) can artichoke hearts, drained and quartered

Ingredients for the wet mix:

- 1 cup almond flour
- Salt and black pepper, to taste
- 1 cup coconut milk
- ½ teaspoon garlic powder

Ingredients for the Dry Mix:

- 2 cups coconut flour
- ¼ teaspoon of paprika
- Salt, pinch

Directions:

1. Drain and cut the artichokes into a quarter size. Pat dry it with a paper towel.
2. Now, take a bowl and add almond flour, salt, pepper, coconut milk, and garlic powder. In a separate small bowl, add all the dry mix ingredients.
3. Now dip artichokes in wet ingredients and then in dry ones.
4. Once all the artichokes are finely coated, layer them onto an air fryer basket lined with parchment paper. Bake it at 400 ° F (205°C) for 18 minutes. Once all the artichokes are done, serve.

Per serving:

Calories 243 | Total Fat 18.8g 24% | Total Carbohydrate 14.8g 5% | Dietary Fiber 8.4g 30% | Protein 5.8g

Cauliflower Bites

Prep: 15 Minutes | Cook Time: 20 Minutes | Makes: 4 Servings

Ingredients:

- 1 Cauliflower florets, cut into bite-size pieces
- ½ tablespoon avocado oil
- 1 tablespoon arrowroot powder
- 1 teaspoon cumin
- Salt, to taste
- 1 cup grated parmesan cheese

Directions:

1. Add cauliflower, avocado oil, arrowroot powder, cumin, and salt, and mix well.
2. Add it to an air fryer basket lined with parchment paper. Air fry it at 390 ° F (200°C) for 20 minutes. Serve with a sprinkle of grate cheese on top.

Per serving:

Calories 180 |Total Fat 9.9g 13% | Total Carbohydrate 9.6g 4%|Dietary Fiber 3.9g 14%|Total Sugars 3.5g |Protein 16.5g

Mushroom Pizzas

Prep: 22 Minutes | Cook Time: 6 Minutes | Makes: 2 Servings

Ingredients:

- 6 large Portobello mushrooms
- Salt and black pepper
- ½ tablespoon of balsamic vinegar
- 4 tablespoons pasta sauce
- 2 cloves of garlic, minced
- 2 olives kalamata olives, chopped
- 2 tablespoons red bell pepper, chopped
- 1 cup parmesan cheese, grated and for topping

Directions:

1. Preheat the air fryer first for 5 minutes at 400 ° F (205°C). Now wash the mushrooms and cut the stem of the mushrooms. Pat dry the mushrooms with a paper towel. Season the mushrooms with salt and pepper. Then toss it with the vinegar.
2. Line an air fryer basket with parchment paper and add mushrooms. Add it to the air fryer and bake for 4 minutes at 400 ° F (205°C). Meanwhile, combine pasta sauce, garlic, olives, salt, black pepper, and bell peppers. Take out the mushrooms. Spoon the mixture over each mushroom. Then toss cheese on top and air fry it for 2more more minutes at 400 ° F (205°C).Plate and serve.

Per serving

Calories 435 | Total Fat 24.5g 31% | Total Carbohydrate 24.8g 9% | Dietary Fiber 5.7g 20% | Protein 33.8g

Cheese Balls

Prep: 20 minutes | cook time: 8 minutes | makes: 2 servings

Ingredients:

- 1 cup almond flour
- 1 cup mozzarella cheese, cubed
- 2 cups ricotta

Directions:

1. Add almond flour to one bowl and mozzarella cubes to another. Add ricotta cheese to a muslin cloth and press out as much water as possible. Make small balls of ricotta cheese using your hands. Then flatten into the palm, and fill the cavity with mozzarella cheese cubes. Then roll into a tight round ball. Roll that ball into the almond flour.
2. Add ricotta balls to the air fryer basket lined with parchment paper. Air fry it for about 8 minutes, flipping halfway through at 400 ° F (205°C). Once done, serve.

Per serving:

Calories 231| Total Fat 14.6g 19%| Total Carbohydrate 8.1g 3%| Dietary Fiber 0.8g 3%| Protein 17.6g

— Halloumi Cheese —

Prep: 12 Minutes | Cook Time: 7-10 Minutes | Makes: 3 Servings

Ingredients:

- 1 pound (450gr) halloumi cheese (cut into slices)
- 2 tablespoons olive oil

Directions:

1. Meanwhile, take a bowl and add cheese and olive oil. Toss it well. Layer the air fryer basket with parchment paper.
2. Add the cheese to the air fryer basket and add the basket to the unit. Air fry them for about 7 - 10 minutes at 400 ° F (205°C)   until they turn golden brown. Add 1-2 more minutes if not crispy. Enjoy.

Per serving:

Calories 261 | Total Fat 18.1g 23% | Total Carbohydrate 19.7g 7% | Dietary Fiber 1.2g 4% | Protein 5g

— Easy Ratatouille —

Prep: 12 Minutes | Cook Time: 8-12 Minutes | Makes: 2 Servings

Ingredients:

- 1 medium eggplant
- 2 small zucchinis
- 2 medium tomatoes
- 1 yellow bell pepper
- 1 red bell pepper
- ½ medium-sized onions
- 1 teaspoon cayenne pepper
- Few sprigs basil
- 4 sprigs oregano
- 4 garlic cloves
- Salt and black pepper, to taste
- 2 tablespoons olive oil
- 2 tablespoons white wine
- 2 teaspoons vinegar

Directions:

1. Start by preheating the air fryer to around 350 ° F (180°C). Slice all the vegetables and add them to a medium bowl. Add the remaining listed ingredients to the bowl and toss.
2. Prepare the basket of air fryers by lining it with parchment paper. Then shift everything to the basket. Set the mode to air frying. Set the timer to around 8 to 12 minutes. Set the temperature to 400 ° F (205°C)
3. Toss the vegetables in the basket once to ensure an even cook. When done, serve and enjoy.

Per serving:

Calories 142 | Total Fat 8g 10% | Total Carbohydrate 16.9g 6% | Dietary Fiber 6.6g 23% | Protein 3.3g

— Easy Pickles —

Prep: 15 Minutes | Cook Time: 10 Minutes | Makes: 4 Servings

Ingredients:

- 20 dill pickle slices
- ½ cup almond flour
- Salt, to taste
- 2eggs (lightly beaten)
- 2 tablespoons dill pickle juice
- ½ teaspoon garlic powder
- ½ teaspoon cayenne pepper
- 2 cups keto bread crumbs
- Oil spray for greasing

Directions:

1. Pat dries the pickles with a paper towel. Add the almond flour and salt to a medium bowl, and set aside. Whisk the egg in a separate bowl.
2. Add dill pickle juice to eggs along with garlic powder and cayenne pepper. Mix it well.
3. Take an air fryer basket and line it with parchment paper. Add the pickles egg wash, then coat with keto bread crumbs. Next, layer it to the basket of the air fryer in a single layer and mist it with oil spray.
4. Add these pickles to the air fryer basket and add the basket to the unit. Air fry the pickles for 8 to 10 minutes at 400 ° F (205°C) . Serve.

Per serving:

Calories 58 | Total Fat 4.2g 5% | Total Carbohydrate 2.1g 1% | Dietary Fiber 0.9g 3% | Protein 3.7g

— Asparagus Frittata —

Prep: 15 Minutes | Cook Time: 10 Minutes| Makes: 2 Servings

Ingredients:

- 2 tablespoons almond milk
- 2 eggs, whisked
- 1/3 cup parmesan cheese, grated
- Salt and black pepper (to taste)
- 6 Asparagus tips, stemmed
- Oil spray for greasing

Directions:

1. Take a bowl and add almond milk, eggs, and cheese. Whisk all the ingredients well. Now season it with salt and black pepper. Add in the asparagus. Pour this egg mixture into an air fryer-safe dish.
2. Add dish to air fryer basket. Air fry it at 390 ° F (200°C)   for 10 minutes. When the eggs are firm, serve.

Per serving:

Calories 245 | Total Fat 17.2g 22% | Total Carbohydrate 4.2g 2% | Dietary Fiber 0.8g 3%| Protein 20.4g

— Saucy Tofu —

Prep: 12 Minutes | Cook Time: 16-18 Minutes | Makes: 2 Servings

Ingredients:
- 1 pound (450gr) super-firm tofu
- 2 tablespoons of tamari sauce
- 2 teaspoons of arrowroot powder

Garlic Sesame Sauce
- 2 garlic cloves, minced
- 2 tablespoons sesame oil
- 2 tablespoons tamari sauce
- 2 teaspoons sesame seeds

Directions:
1. Preheat the air fryer for 7 minutes at 300 ° F (150°C). Drain and press the tofu and cut it into small cubes. Add the tofu to the bowl and toss with tamari sauce and arrowroot powder. Set it aside. Set the sauce ingredients aside as well.
2. Take an air fryer basket and line it with parchment paper. Add the tofu cube to the basket and add the basket to the unit. Air fry it for 12 minutes at 400 ° F (205°C)
3. Meanwhile, stir fry garlic in sesame oil using a skillet for 2 minutes. Then add it to a bowl. To the garlic, add sesame seeds and tamari sauce. Once the tofu is ready, serve it with the prepared sauce. Then serve hot.

Per serving:
Calories 471 | Total Fat 34.9g 45% | Total Carbohydrate 11.4g 4% | Dietary Fiber 5.6g 20% | Protein 36.5g

— Crumbed Asparagus —

Prep: 15 Minutes | Cook Time: 5 Minutes | Makes: 2 Servings

Ingredients:
- 2 eggs, 1 cup almond flour
- ¼ cup pork rinds, grated
- 12 asparagus (cut in half)

Directions:
1. Crack eggs in a bowl and whisk them well. Next, take a separate bowl and add almond flour with pork rinds. Mix it well. Now coat the asparagus with egg, then dip in flour. Add the asparagus to the basket of air fryers lined with parchment paper.Cook it at 390 ° F (200°C) for 5 minutes. Serve and enjoy.

Per serving:
Calories 172 | Total Fat 12.1g 16% | Total Carbohydrate 7.1g 3% | Dietary Fiber 3.5g 13% | Protein 11.8g

— Crispy Jicama Fries —

Prep: 20 Minutes | Cook Time: 12-24 Minutes | Makes: 2 Servings

Ingredients:
- 4 cups jicama (peeled and cut ½ inch (12mm) thick)
- 1 tablespoon olive oil
- ½ teaspoon garlic powder
- ½ teaspoon cumin, Salt and black pepper, to taste

Directions:
1. Take a large pot and boil water in it over a medium flame. Add the jicama to the water and cook for 18 to 25 minutes. Next, take it out for water and pat it dry with a paper towel. Now preheat the air fryer to 400 ° F (205°C) for 4 minutes
2. Take a bowl and jicama with olive oil, garlic powder, cumin, salt, and black pepper. Toss it well.
3. Layer the parchment paper onto the air fryer basket. Work in batches and add the jicama into the air fryer. Air fry it for 12 minutes at 400 ° F (205°C). Repeat for the remaining fries.

Per serving:
Calories 156 | Total Fat 7.4g 9% | Total Carbohydrate 21.9g 8% |Dietary Fiber 11.9g 43% | Protein 2g

— Cheese Balls —

Prep: 12 Minutes | Cook Time: 12 Minutes | Makes: 2 Serving

Ingredients:
- ½ cup feta cheese, crumbled
- 2/3 cup Gouda cheese, shredded
- ½ cup almond flour
- 2 tablespoons mint leaves, chopped
- 1 tablespoon dried oregano
- 2 eggs
- ½ cup Parmesan cheese
- ½ cup pork rinds, grated, oil spray

Directions:
1. Combine feta cheese, Gouda cheese, almond flour, mint, and oregano in a bowl. Mix it well, add egg, and incorporate all the ingredients. Add parmesan cheese with pork rinds in a separate bowl and make small balls of the cheese batter and roll them in the cheese and pork rinds. Mist it with oil spray.
2. Add it to an air fryer basket lined with parchment paper. Add the basket to the unit. Close the unit. Air fry it at 390 ° F (200°C) for 12 minutes, shaking the basket halfway through. Serve and enjoy.

Per serving:
Calories 704 | Total Fat 51g 65% | Total Carbohydrate 8.3g 3% | Dietary Fiber 2.1g 8% | Protein 56.3g

— Chicken Strips —

Prep: 22 Minutes | Cook Time: 16 Minutes | Makes: 6 Servings

Ingredients:

- ½ cup coconut flour
- 2 eggs, whisked
- 1 cup parmesan cheese
- ½ cup almond flour
- 1 teaspoon smoked paprika
- 1 teaspoon black pepper
- 6 chicken breast strips
- Salt and pepper, to taste

Directions:

1. Add coconut flour to a bowl and set aside. Whisk eggs in a separate bowl. In the third bowl, combine parmesan cheese, almond flour, paprika, salt, and black pepper. Coat the chicken with coconut flour, then dip into egg and finally into cheese mixture.
2. Add the strips to the basket lined with parchment paper. Air fry it for 16 minutes at 400 ° F (205°C). Serve and enjoy.

Per serving:

Calories 363 | Total Fat 16.4g 21% | Total Carbohydrate 22.1g 8% | Dietary Fiber 5.5g 20% | Protein 30.5g

— Easy Spinach —

Prep: 10 Minutes | Cook Time: 8-10 Minutes | Makes: 2 Servings

Ingredients:

- 6 ounces (170gr) of fresh spinach leaves
- Few pinches of sea salt
- 2 tablespoons of olive oil for greasing
- oil spray for greasing

Directions:

1. Preheat the air fryer for 4 minutes at high. Take a large bowl and add washed spinal leaves to it. Then pat dry the spinach leaves with a paper towel. Roll the towel so the leaves get dry completely. Take a large bowl and add sea salt and olive oil. Toss the dry leaves in it.
2. Grease an air fryer basket with oil spray. Add spinach leaves into the air fryer basket to avoid overlapping. Air fry it for 8 minutes at 400 ° F (205°C).
3. Toss after 4 minutes of cooking. If the leaves are not crispy, air fry for 1-2 more minutes. Once it's done, serve.

Per serving:

Calories 142 | Total Fat 14.6g 19% | Total Carbohydrate 3.1g 1% | Dietary Fiber 1.9g 7% | Protein 2.4g

— Simple Chicken Wings —

Prep: 12 Minutes | Cook Time: 16 -18 Minutes | Makes: 2 Servings

Ingredients:

- 10 chicken wings
- 4 teaspoon avocado oil
- salt and black pepper, to taste
- 1 tablespoon spicy zaatar
- 1/3 cup of Tabasco original red sauce

Directions:

1. Pat dry the chicken wings with a paper towel and add to a large bowl. Toss it with avocado oil, salt, pepper, and zaatar seasoning. Mix well so the wings coat.
2. Take an air fryer basket and line it with parchment paper. Put the wings in a single layer inside the air fryer basket. Add the basket to the unit. Cook it at 400 ° F (205°C) for 16-18 minutes, depending upon the size of the wings.
3. Flip the wings halfway through. Once done, serve with sauce. Enjoy hot.

Per serving:

Calories 1400 | Total Fat 55.3g 71% | Total Carbohydrate 0.6g 0% | Dietary Fiber 0.4g 2% | Protein 211.3g

— Simple Beef Kebab —

Prep: 15 Minutes | Cook Time: 10 -12Minutes | Makes: 2 Servings

Ingredients:

- 1 pound (450gr) ground beef
- 1 large white onion, chopped
- 2 tablespoons cilantro, chopped
- 1 teaspoon chili powder
- 1 teaspoon coriander, ground
- Salt and pepper, to taste
- oil spray for misting

Directions:

1. Take wooden skewers and soak them in water. Meanwhile, take a bowl and add beef with the remaining listed ingredients. Mix well, so the ingredients combine. Take out the wooden skewers and pat them dry with a paper towel. They skewed the meat onto skewers in the shape of kebabs. Mist the kebabs with oil spray.
2. Add it to an air fryer basket lined with parchment paper. Add the basket to the unit. Cook it at 400 ° F (205°C) for 10-12 minutes, rotating halfway through. Once done, serve.

Per serving:

Calories 458 | Total Fat 14.7g 19% | Total Carbohydrate 7.8g 3% | Dietary Fiber 2.1g 7% | Protein 69.8g

Meaty Eggplants

Prep: 25 Minutes | Cook Time: 40 Minutes | Makes: 4 Servings

Ingredients:

- 1 tablespoon of olive oil
- ¼ cup spring onion
- ½ cup marinara sauce
- 1 teaspoon ginger garlic paste
- Salt to taste
- ½ teaspoon of red chili powder
- ½ cup beef meat, grounded
- 2 medium eggplants
- 1 cup parmesan cheese

Directions:

1. Prepare the filling by heating the oil in a cooking pan and sauté onion for 2 minutes. Then add marinara sauce and ginger garlic paste. Cook for 2 minutes, and then add salt and red chili powder. Then add meat and let it cook for 10 minutes.
2. Remove the eggplant green part and center core it. Add meat to the eggplant.
3. Add the eggplant to the basket of air fryers lined with parchment paper. Add an air fryer basket to the unit and close it. Air fry it for 20 minutes at 400 ° F (205°C) Once 15 minutes pass, take out the eggplants and top with equally distributed parmesan cheese. Once it's done, serve.

Per serving:

Calories 281 | Total Fat 14.5g 19% | Total Carbohydrate 22.4g 8% | Dietary Fiber 10.6g 38% | Protein 19.7g

Pork Bites

Prep: 12 Minutes | Cook Time: 12 Minutes | Makes: 2 Servings

Ingredients:

- 1 pound (450gr) pork tenderloin
- 4 teaspoons of olive oil
- 1 tablespoon Cajun seasoning

Directions:

1. Start by preheating the air fryer to around 390 ° F (200°C). Take the pork tenderloin and slice it into smaller pieces, coating each piece with oil and seasoning it with Cajun seasoning.
2. Next, place parchment paper over the basket of the air fryer. Select bake mode. Adjust the time to 12 minutes. Adjust the temperature to 400 ° F (205°C), and add the tenderloin pieces into the air fryer basket. Close the basket and let it air fry. Once the pork becomes nice and crispy, take it out, and serve.

Per serving:

Calories 404 | Total Fat 17.3g 22% | Total Carbohydrate 0g 0% | Dietary Fiber 0% | Protein 59.4g

Eggs Omelet with Tuna Fish and Avocados

Prep: 12 Minutes | Cook Time: 6-8 Minutes | Makes: 2 Servings

Ingredients:

- 6 eggs, beaten
- 1 red tomato, diced
- Pinch of sea salt
- ½ pound (230gr) tuna fish, diced
- 1 avocado, diced

Directions:

1. Take a bowl and crack eggs in it. Then add diced tomatoes, sea salt, and tuna pieces. Mix it well. Grease a cake pan with oil spray. Pour the egg batter into the pan.
2. Add the cake pan to the basket. Add the air fryer basket to the unit. Cook at 350 ° F (180°C) for 6 -8 minutes at high.
3. Once the eggs get firm, take them out, and serve them with slices of avocado. Serve and enjoy.

Per serving:

Calories 430 | Total Fat 34.3g 44% | Total Carbohydrate 14.1g 5% | Dietary Fiber 7.7g 28% | Protein 20.8g

Greek Pork

Prep: 7 Minutes | Cook Time: 22 Minutes | Makes: 2 Servings

Ingredients:

- 16 ounces (450gr) of pork tenderloin
- 2 tablespoons olive oil
- 3 teaspoons red wine vinegar
- 2 teaspoons of garlic, minced
- salt and pepper, to taste
- ½ teaspoon dill, dried
- 4 ounces (115gr) of tzatziki sauce
- 6 lettuce leaves
- 2 cucumbers, diced
- 2 tomatoes, diced
- 2ounces (60gr) Kalamata olives
- 6 ounces (170gr) feta cheese, crumbled

Directions:

1. Start by drizzling the pork with olive oil, vinegar, garlic, salt, and pepper. Make sure to message on the tenderloin to ensure it is seasoned.
2. Put the tenderloin in the air fryer basket, and set the time to 22 minutes. Set the temperature to 400 ° F (205°C)..
3. Layer the lettuce leaves first with tzatziki sauce, followed by cucumber, tomatoes, olive, and feta cheese. Then add the cooked tenderloin and serve.

Per serving:

Calories 434 | Total Fat 25.9g 33% | Total Carbohydrate 13.3g 5% | Dietary Fiber 2.1g 7% | Protein 37.5g

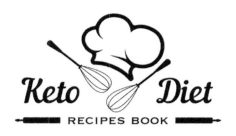

Chapter

6

Appetizers and Snacks

— Spicy Cheesy Cauliflower —

Prep: 15 Minutes | Cook Time: 16 Minutes | Makes: 2 Servings

Ingredients:

- ¼ tablespoon of cumin seeds
- ½ teaspoon of coriander seeds
- Sea salt, to taste
- Black pepper, to taste
- ¼teaspoon of red pepper
- ¼ teaspoon of Turmeric
- ½ cup shredded Mozzarella cheese
- ½ cup shredded sharp cheddar cheese
- 1 medium cauliflower, cut into florets

Directions:

1. Preheat the air fryer to 400 ° F (205°C) before starting the cooking. Add cumin, coriander, salt, pepper, red pepper, Turmeric, mozzarella cheese, and sharp cheddar cheese. Dust the cauliflower florets well with spice and cheese mix.
2. Add the florets inside the air fryer basket. Air fry it for 16 minutes at 400 ° F (205°C), tossing it halfway through. Once it's done, serve.

Per serving:

Calories 248 | Total Fat 11.3g 14% | Total Carbohydrate 24.5g 9% | Dietary Fiber 10.9g 39% | Protein 17.7g

— Snack Time Stuffed Zucchini —

Prep: 12 Minutes | Cook Time: 20 Minutes | Makes: 2 Servings

Ingredients:

- 2 medium zucchinis
- 4 tablespoons butter
- ¼ cup onion, chopped
- ½ Red bell pepper, chopped
- 2 pork sausages, crumbled
- ¼ teaspoon ground fennel seed
- Salt and black pepper, to taste
- 1 oregano spring
- 2 cups mozzarella cheese, shredded

Directions:

1. Peel the zucchini and cut it lengthwise. Scoop the cavity of zucchinis.
2. Melt butter in a skillet and cook onions for 4 minutes at low. Then add the red bell pepper, crumbled sausages, fennel seeds, salt, pepper, and oregano, and cook for 10 minutes at low. Once the meat gets brown, fill the cavity of the zucchinis with the meat mixture. Add on top the shredded cheese.
3. Put it in an air fryer basket lined with parchment paper. Air fry it at 375 ° F (190°C) for 14-16 minutes. Once it's done, serve and enjoy.

Per serving:

Calories 374 | Total Fat 32.2g 41% | Total Carbohydrate 11.2g 4% | Dietary Fiber 2.9g 10% | Protein 13.6g

— Cheese Filled Mushrooms —

Prep: 16 Minutes | Cook Time: 8 Minutes | Makes: 2 Servings

Ingredients:

- 10 ounces (280gr) fresh mushrooms
- 6 ounces (170gr) of cream cheese
- ½ cup parmesan cheese, shredded
- 1/6 cup cheddar cheese, shredded sharp
- 1/6 cup cheddar cheese, shredded white
- 1 teaspoon Worcestershire sauce
- 2 garlic cloves Minced
- Salt and pepper to taste

Directions:

1. Cut the mushroom stem so it is prepared for stuffing. Now chop the stems of mushrooms and add them to a bowl. Use soft cream cheese and add to stems.
2. Then add parmesan, sharp cheddar, cheddar white, Worcestershire sauce, garlic clove, salt, and pepper. Mix it well and stuff the mushrooms with it.
3. Put it in an air fryer basket lined with parchment paper. Air Fry it for 8 minutes at 380 ° F (195°C). Once done, serve.

Per serving:

Calories 585 | Total Fat 48.2g 62 %Total Carbohydrate 9.9g 4% | Dietary Fiber 1.4g 5% |Protein 33.6g

— Cauliflower tots —

Prep: 10 Minutes | Cook Time: 6-8 Minutes | Makes: 6 Servings

Ingredients:

- 4 cups cauliflower
- 1 egg beaten lightly
- ½ cup almond flour
- 1 cup cheddar cheese shredded
- 1 cup parmesan cheese shredded or grated
- 2 tablespoons Italian seasonings
- Oil spray for greasing

Directions:

1. Steam the cauliflower florets using a steamer for 3 minutes, then set aside. Then pulse it inside the food processor. Take it out in a bowl and add egg and mix well. Then add the almond flour. Remix it and add cheddar cheese, parmesan cheese, and Italian seasoning. Mix well and form tots.
2. Mist the tots with oil spray.
3. Layer the tots onto the air fryer basket. Air fry at 400 ° F (205°C) for 6-8 minutes, flipping halfway. Once it's done, serve.

Per serving:

Calories 222 | Total Fat 10.4g 13% | Total Carbohydrate 26.4g 10% | Dietary Fiber 3g 11% |Protein 7.7g

— Simple Tempeh —

Prep: 10 Minutes | Cook Time: 14 Minutes | Makes: 2 Servings

Ingredients:

- 10 ounces (280gr) of Tempeh, sliced into ½ inches
- 2 tablespoons avocado oil
- 1 tablespoon coconut aminos
- 2 teaspoons toasted sesame oil
- Pink salt, to taste
- ½ teaspoon garlic powder

Directions:

1. Preheat the air fryer to 400 ° F (205°C) before starting the cooking. Slice the Tempeh into ½ inch cubes. Put it in a bowl and add avocado oil, coconut amnion, sesame oil, salt, and garlic powder. Let it sit for 10 minutes.
2. Now add the Tempeh to the air fryer basket lined with parchment paper. Air fry it at 390 ° F (200°C) for 14 minutes. Once it's crispy and golden, serve.

Per serving:

Calories 335 | Total Fat 21.6g 28% | Total Carbohydrate 14.6g 5% | Dietary Fiber 0.7g 2% | Protein 26.6g

— Beef Jerky —

Prep: 12 Minutes | Cook Time: 2 hours | Makes: 4 Servings

Ingredients:

- 2 pounds (900gr) flank steak, strip cut
- 4 tablespoons stevia
- 6 tablespoons soy sauce or coconut amino
- 2 tablespoons chili garlic sauce
- 2 tablespoons tomato paste
- 2 tablespoons water
- Oil spray for greasing

Directions:

1. Take a freezer bag and add flank steak inside a freezer in it for 2 hours. Then, once solid, slice it into jerky pieces against the grain. Now combine all the remaining listed ingredients in a bowl. Marinate the strips of meat inside it overnight by placing it in a refrigerator. Remove the strips of meat from the marinade.
2. Now grease an air fryer basket with oil spray. Place strips inside the air fryer basket in a single layer. Air fries it at 200 ° F (95°C) for 2 hours. Once dark in color and dried out, the jerky is done. Let it rest for 10 minutes, then serve.

Per serving:

Calories 448 | Total Fat 19.1g 24% | Total Carbohydrate 1.5g 1% | Dietary Fiber 0.3g 1% | Protein 63.5g

— Sausage Bacon Bi —

Prep: 10 Minutes | Cook Time: 15-20 Minutes | Makes: 2 Servings

Ingredients:

- 1 pound (450gr) bacon strips
- 12 ounces (340gr) sausage links, cooked and thawed
- ½ cup stevia for coating

Directions:

1. Cut bacon strips and sausage links in half. Wrap the sausage links with bacon strips. Roll it in stevia coating. Put it in an air fryer basket lined with parchment paper. Work in a single layer and batches.
2. Air fry it for 15-20 minutes at 325 ° F (160°C). Flip the sausages halfway. Once done, serve.

Per serving:

Calories 295 | Total Fat 26.5g 34% | Total Carbohydrate 2g 1% | Dietary Fiber 0g 0% | Protein 11.4g

— Onion Fritter —

Prep: 20 Minutes | Cook Time: 10 Minutes | Makes: 4 Servings

Mint Sauce Ingredients:

- 1 cup Greek yogurt
- 1 tablespoon of mint, fresh
- 4 tablespoons of coriander leaves,
- Salt, to taste
- 1 green chili
- Black pepper, to taste
- ½ teaspoon of dry pomegranate seeds

Onion Fritter Ingredients:

- 1 cup gram flour
- 2 onions medium, peeled, and thinly sliced
- 1 teaspoon of coriander seeds of crushed
- 1 teaspoon red chili powder
- ¼teaspoon turmeric powder
- ¼teaspoon baking soda, Salt, to taste

Directions:

1. Combine all the sauce ingredients in a blender, and then set aside for further use. Preheat the air fryer to 390 ° F (200°C) for 3 minutes. Line an air fryer basket with parchment paper and grease the paper with oil spray.
2. Take a bowl and add the entire onion fritter ingredients to it. Let it sit for 10 minutes. Use a spoon and drop the mixture on to air fryer basket.
3. Air fry it for 10 minutes at 390 ° F (200°C), flipping halfway. Serve it with prepared mint sauce.

Per serving:

Calories 289 | Total Fat 4.9g 6% | Total Carbohydrate 28.6g 10% | Dietary Fiber 3.8g 14% | Protein 31.2g

— Crab Cake Fritters —

Prep: 15 Minutes | Cook Time: 12 Minutes | Makes: 2 Servings

Ingredients:

- 12 ounces (340gr) of crab meat
- 6 tablespoons of pork rinds, grated
- Salt and pepper, to taste
- 2 large organic eggs
- dash of paprika

Directions:

1. Preheat the air fryer to 390 ° F (205°C) for 4 minutes before starting the cooking process. Add all the ingredients in a bowl and make fritter shapes. Mist the fritter with oil spray.
2. Add the fritter to the air fryer basket lined with parchment paper. Air fry it for 12 minutes at 350 ° F (180°C), flipping halfway through. Once it's crispy and golden, take it out. Serve and enjoy.

Per serving:

Calories 304 | Total Fat 9.1g 12% | Total Carbohydrate 18g 7% | Dietary Fiber 0.9g 3% | Protein 30.3g

Turkey Cutlets with Mushroom Sauce

Prep: 10 Minutes | Cook Time: 12 Minutes | Makes: 4 Servings

Ingredients:

- 1.5 pounds (680gr) of turkey, ground
- 2 tablespoons avocado oil
- Salt and black pepper, to taste
- Oil spray for greasing

Mushroom Sauce:

- 1 cup coconut milk
- 1 cup heavy cream
- ½ cup chopped mushroom
- Salt and black pepper, to taste
- ½ cup parmesan cheese, grated

Directions:

1. Preheat your air fryer before cooking to 400 ° F (205°C). Add turkey meat, avocado oil, salt, and black pepper in a bowl and mix well. Make small patties and mist the patties with oil spray.
2. Put it in an air fryer basket lined with parchment paper. Air fry it for 12 minutes at 390 ° F (200°C).. Flip the patties halfway through.
3. Meanwhile, simmer coconut milk, cream, mushrooms, salt, pepper, and parmesan cheese in a saucepan. Once thick, serve with patties.

Per serving:

Calories 633 | Total Fat 41g 53% | Total Carbohydrate 5.9g 2% | Dietary Fiber 1.7g 6% | Protein 61.2g

— Parmesan Brussels sprouts —

Prep: 15 Minutes | Cook Time: 10 Minutes | Makes: 2 Servings

Ingredients:

- 1 pound (450gr) Brussels sprouts, ends trimmed
- 1 teaspoon garlic powder
- Salt and black pepper, to taste
- ½ cup pork rinds, grated
- ½ cup Parmesan cheese, grated

Directions:

1. Add Brussels sprouts, garlic powder, salt, and black pepper into a large bowl. Then mix it well. Put it in the air fryer basket and then air fry it for 6 minutes at 400 ° F (205°C). Halfway through, stir the Brussels sprouts. Then sprinkle parmesan cheese and pork rinds on top. Air fry for 4 more minutes. Once it's crispy, serve.

Per serving:

Calories 443 | Total Fat 22.8g 29% | Total Carbohydrate 23.7g 9% | Dietary Fiber 8.7g 31% | Protein 44g

Coconut Shrimp and Apricot Sauce —

Prep: 10 Minutes | Cook Time: 4-6 Minutes | Makes: 4 Servings

Ingredients:

- 1 cup coconut flakes, unsweetened shredded
- ½ cup pork rind
- 2 large eggs
- 2 dashes of hot sauce
- salt and black pepper, to taste
- 20 shrimps, cleaned, deveined, and peeled

Sauce Ingredients:

- ¼ cup apricot preserves
- 1 teaspoon apple cider vinegar
- ½ teaspoon crushed red pepper flakes

Directions:

1. Preheat the air fryer for 6 minutes at 400 ° F (205°C) before starting the cooking. Take a bowl and add coconut flakes and pork rinds. In a separate bowl, whisk eggs and add hot sauce, salt, and black pepper. Whisk the eggs well.
2. Dip the shrimp into the egg mixture, and then coat it with coconut flakes and pork rinds.
3. Air fry it for 4-6 minutes at 400 ° F (205°C), flipping halfway. Meanwhile, add all the sauce ingredients to a saucepan and simmer at low for 5 minutes. Add shrimp to the sauce and toss to coat, then serve.

Per serving:

Calories 322 | Total Fat 9.6g 12% | Total Carbohydrate 21.4g 8% | Dietary Fiber 0.2g 1% | Protein 37.5g

— Spicy Chicken Jerky —

Prep: 25 Minutes | Cook Time: 25-30 Minutes | Makes: 1-2 Servings

Ingredients:

- 6 ounces (170gr) of chicken breasts, cut into thin strips
- 1 teaspoon of garlic powder
- 1 teaspoon of onion powder
- 1 teaspoon of lemon pepper
- 2 teaspoons Cajun seasoning

Directions:

1. Rub the boneless chicken breast strips with all the listed spices. Put it in an air fryer basket lined with parch met paper. Air fry it for 10 minutes at 200 ° F (95°C).
2. Then thread the strip into wooden skewers and Put it in the air fryer basket again. Air fry it for 25-30 minutes at 370 ° F (190°C).
3. Once the jerky is ready, remove the strip and let it get cool. Then serve.

Per serving:

Calories 173 | Total Fat 6.4g 8% | Total Carbohydrate 2.7g 1% | Dietary Fiber 0.5g 2% | Protein 25.1g

— Boneless Wings —

Prep: 20 Minutes | Cook Time: 8-10 Minutes | Makes: 4 Servings

Ingredients:

- 2 pounds (900gr) of chicken breast, boneless skinless, and cubed into small pieces
- 2 teaspoons paprika
- 1 teaspoon garlic powder
- 2 teaspoons onion powder
- Salt and black pepper, to taste
- 1 cup buffalo sauce, sugar-free keto-based

Side serving:

- 1 cup blue cheese dressing

Directions:

1. Preheat the air fryer to 390 ° F (200°C) before starting the cooking process. Pat dries the chicken breast pieces. Season the chicken breast pieces with paprika, garlic powder, onion powder, salt, pepper, and buffalo sauce.
2. Put it in an air fryer basket lined with parchment paper. Air fry it for 8 to 10 minutes at 350 ° F, flipping halfway. Once the internal temperature is 165 ° F (75°C), take out the cubes. Serve with blue cheese dressing.

Per serving:

Calories 577 | Total Fat 37.9g 49% | Total Carbohydrate 6.6g 2% | Dietary Fiber 0.5g 2% | Protein 51.4g

— Mini Pepper Nachos —

Prep: 15 Minutes | Cook Time: 14 Minutes | Makes: 4 Servings

Ingredients:
- 2 teaspoons of butter
- 1 pound (450gr) ground beef, browned and drained
- 1 tablespoon taco seasoning
- 2-4 tablespoons water
- 4 baby bell peppers, halved and seeded
- 1 cup shredded fiesta blend cheese

Optional Topping Ideas:
- ¼ cup chopped cilantro
- ¼ cup sliced black olives
- ½ cup Sour Cream

Directions:
1. Preheat the air fryer to 390 ° F (200°C) before starting the cooking process. Take a skillet, add butter and ground beef, and cook at medium heat. Add taco seasoning and mix well; add a bit of water if the meat gets dry, and start sticking to the skillet. Remove seeds from the center of bell peppers. Add the meat inside the cavity of the bell pepper. To the top of each bell pepper, sprinkle an equal amount of fiesta blend cheese.
2. Add the peppers to the air fryer basket greased with oil spray. Air fry it for 10 to 14 minutes at 360 ° F (180°C). Serve with listed additional toppings.

Per serving:

Calories 413 | Total Fat 25.3g 32% | Total Carbohydrate 2.2g 1% | Fiber 0.3g 1% | Protein 42.5g

— Cheese Puffs —

Prep: 10 Minutes | Cook Time: 5 Minutes | Makes: 2 Servings

Ingredients:
- 4 ounces (115gr) of cheese, personal choice preferred

Directions:
1. Preheat the air fryer to 390 ° F before starting the cooking process. Cut the cheese into ¼ inch pieces. Lay the cheese pieces onto a paper towel and cover with one more paper towel. Place it inside the fridge for 2 hours. Take it out and Put it in a single layer inside the air fryer lined with parchment paper. Air fry it for 5 minutes at 390 ° F (200°C). Once done, let it cool. Serve, and enjoy.

Per serving:

Calories 229 | Total Fat 18.8g 24% | Total Carbohydrate 0.7g 0% | Dietary Fiber 0g 0% | Protein 14.1g

— Pork Jerky —

Prep: 10 Minutes | Cook Time: 120 Minutes | Makes: 4 Servings

Ingredients:
- 2 pounds (900gr) of ground pork
- 2 tablespoons sesame oil
- 1 tablespoon Sriracha
- 1 tablespoon coconut amino
- 1 tablespoon balsamic vinegar
- Salt and black pepper, pinch
- 1 teaspoon onion powder
- ½ teaspoon pink curing salt

Directions:
1. Combine pork, oil, Sriracha, coconut amino, vinegar, salt and pepper, onion powder, and pink curing salt in a bowl and refrigerate overnight.
2. Take a jerky gun, and form as much meat jerky on to air fryer basket lined with parchment paper.
3. Air fry it at 150 ° F (65°C) for 1 hour. Flip and cook for 1 more hour
4. Take the jerky out and cover it with a paper towel. Let it dry overnight. Then serve it anytime as a little snack.

Per serving:

Calories 391 | Total Fat 14.8g 19% | Total Carbohydrate 1.3g 0% | Dietary Fiber 0g 0% | Protein 59.4g

— Zesty Balsamic Veggies —

Prep: 12 Minutes | Cook Time: 6 Minutes | Makes: 4 Servings

Ingredients:
- 2 avocados, pitted
- 6 plum tomatoes (diced)
- ½ cup fresh basil, diced
- ¼cup cheddar cheese
- 2 teaspoons minced garlic
- 1 tablespoon balsamic vinegar
- 1 tablespoon olive oil

Directions:
1. Pit the avocados and set them aside. Take out the center flesh from the center of avocados to create a cavity. Combine the tomatoes, basil, cheese, garlic, vinegar, and olive oil in a bowl. Mix it well and top it into each avocado cavity.
2. Place each avocado in the air fryer basket lined with parchment paper. Air fry it for 6 minutes at 370 ° F (185°C). Once done, serve.

Per serving:

Calories 309 | Total Fat 25.8g 33% | Total Carbohydrate 18.7g 7% | Dietary Fiber 8.8g 32% | Protein 6.1g

— Mozzarella Sticks —

Prep: 20 Minutes | Cook Time: 8 Minutes | Makes: 4 Servings

Ingredients:
- Oil spray for greasing
- 1/3 cup almond flour
- ¼ teaspoon paprika
- ¼ teaspoon sea salt
- 1 teaspoon Italian seasoning
- ½ teaspoon onion powder
- ½ teaspoon garlic powder
- 2 large eggs
- 6 mozzarella cheese sticks, part-skim
- ½ cup finely crushed pork rinds

Directions:
1. Take an air fryer basket and line it with parchment paper. Then spray the parchment paper with oil spray.
2. Combine the almond flour, paprika, salt, Italian seasoning, onion powder, garlic powder, and pork rinds in a bowl. Whisk eggs in a separate bowl.
3. Cut the mozzarella cheese into thick sticks. Dip it inside the egg and then into the flour mixture. Then coat it with pork rinds,
4. Layer it into an air fryer basket. Air fry it at 375 ° F (190°C) for 8 minutes. Once done, serve.

Per serving:

Calories 182 | Total Fat 12g 15% | Total Carbohydrate 1.4g 1% | Dietary Fiber 0.4g 1% | Protein 17.9g

— Bacon-Wrapped Asparagus —

Prep: 6 Minutes | Cook Time: 10-16 Minutes | Makes: 4 Servings

Ingredients:
- 24 Asparagus spears
- Salt and black pepper, to taste
- 1 teaspoon of paprika
- 2 teaspoons of avocado oil
- 6 Slices bacon, thick

Directions:
1. Pat dries the asparagus and makes a bundle of 4 asparagus each. Season it with salt, pepper, paprika, and avocado oil.
2. Line an air fryer basket with parchment paper. Wrap each asparagus bundle with a thick bacon strip.
3. Add the wrapped asparagus to an air fryer basket lined with parchment paper. Air fry it for 10-16 minutes at 360 ° F (180°C). Once it's cooked, serve.

Per serving:

Calories 188 | Total Fat 12.5g 16% | Total Carbohydrate 6.5g 2% | Dietary Fiber 3.3g 12% | Protein 13.8g

— Crab Sticks —

Prep: 12 Minutes | Cook Time: 6-8 Minutes | Makes: 4 Servings

Ingredients:
- 2 pounds (900gr) of imitation crab leg, peeled
- Cooking spray
- 1 tablespoon Cajun seasoning

Garlic butter sauce:
- 6 tablespoons of butter
- 2 cloves of garlic
- ½ teaspoon of lemon juice
- ¼ cup chopped parsley

Directions:
1. Preheat the air fryer for 6 minutes at 400 ° F (205°C). Cut the crab meat into strips. Mist the crab strips with oil spray—dust with Cajun seasoning.
2. Add to oil greased basket of the air fryer and air fry for 6 minutes at 350 ° F (180°C).
3. Heat butter in a saucepan and add garlic cloves. Cook for 1 minute, and then add lemon Juice and parsley. Cook for 30 seconds and serve with crab.

Per serving:

Calories 358 | Total Fat 17.5g 22% | Total Carbohydrate 28.4g 10% | Dietary Fiber 0.2g 1% | Protein 20.4g

— Pepper Chili Prawns —

Prep: 12 Minutes | Cook Time: 4-6 Minutes | Makes: 2 Servings

Ingredients:
- 12 large Shrimps, deveined and peeled
- 4 eggs
- ¼ teaspoon garlic powder
- ½ teaspoon red Pepper powder
- ½ teaspoon red chili paste
- 1 teaspoon coconut flour
- ½ teaspoon coconut amino
- 1 teaspoon stevia
- 1 teaspoon balsamic vinegar
- Avocado Oil, as needed
- 1 cup pork rinds, grated

Directions:
1. Preheat the air fryer before cooking at 400 ° F (205°C) for 3 minutes. Combine all the ingredients except pork rinds in a bowl. Coat the shrimp with a bowl mixture, then coat with pork rinds.
2. Arrange shrimp in an air fryer basket lined with parchment paper. Air fry the shrimp for 4-6 minutes at 400 ° F (205°C), flipping halfway. Once it is cooked, serve and enjoy!

Per serving:

Calories 618 | Total Fat 44.2g 57% | Total Carbohydrate 11g 4% | Dietary Fiber 7g 25% | Protein 47.7g

⚊ Roasted Nuts ⚊

Prep: 10 Minutes | Cook Time: 20 Minutes | Makes: 4 Servings

Ingredients:

- 1 cup almonds
- 1 cup cashews
- 1 cup peanuts

Directions:

1. Mix all the nuts in a bowl and add to the air fryer basket lined with parchment paper.
2. Air fry it for 20 minutes at 350 ° F (180°C), tossing halfway. Once done, serve.

Per serving:

Calories 541 | Total Fat 45.7g 59% | Total Carbohydrate 22.2g 8% | Dietary Fiber 7.1g 25% | Protein 19.7g

⚊ Cheeseburger Onion Rings ⚊

Prep: 16 Minutes | Cook Time: 12-14 Minutes | Makes: 2 Servings

Ingredients:

- 2 large onions
- 1 pound (450gr) lean ground beef
- 1/3 cup ketchup
- 2 tablespoons mustard
- ¼ teaspoon salt
- 4 ounces (115gr) of cheddar cheese
- 3/4 cup almond flour
- 2 teaspoons garlic powder
- 4 eggs
- 1-½ cups pork rinds, grated
- Oil spray for greasing

Side serving:

- ½ cup mayonnaise

Directions:

1. Preheat the air fryer to 390 ° F (200°C) before starting the cooking process. Cut onions into thick round slices and separate the rings. Add beef, ketchup, mustard, and salt into a bowl and mix well. Fill the larger rings with beef mixture and top each with a small amount of cheese.
2. In a small bowl, mix almond flour and garlic powder. Crack eggs in a separate bowl. Add pork rinds to the third bowl. Dip the filled onions in almond flour, egg, and pork rinds.
3. Layer the onion rings inside the air-fryer basket. Air fry it for 12-14 minutes at 390 ° F (200°C), flipping halfway. Serve once golden with mayonnaise.

Per serving:

Calories 734 | Total Fat 42.7g 55% | Total Carbohydrate 23.9g 9% | Dietary Fiber 3.2g 11 % | Protein 64.7g

⚊ Bacon Wrapped Green Beans ⚊

Prep: 16 Minutes | Cook Time: 10-12 Minutes | Makes: 4 Servings

Ingredients:

- 20 fresh green beans
- 10 slices of uncured bacon
- Salt and black pepper, to taste
- Oil spray for greasing

Directions:

1. Make a bundle of green beans by wrapping two green beans with one bacon strip. Trim the edges of the green beans. Season it with salt and black pepper
2. Put it inside the air fryer basket lined with parchment paper. Mist the bundles with oil spray. Air fry it at 360 ° F (180°C) for 10-12 minutes. Once done, serve.

Per serving:

Calories 125 | Total Fat 4.2g 5% | Total Carbohydrate 20.4g 7% | Dietary Fiber 9.7g 35% | Protein 6.4g

⚊ Coated Mushrooms ⚊

Prep: 10 Minutes | Cook Time: 7 Minutes | Makes: 2 Servings

Ingredients:

- 10 ounces (280gr) of Portobello mushrooms
- ½ cup almond flour
- 4 organic eggs
- 1-2 cups pork rinds
- 1 teaspoon garlic powder
- 2 teaspoons onion powder
- 1 teaspoon smoked paprika
- 1 tablespoon Italian seasoning
- Salt and pepper, a few pinches
- Olive oil spray

Directions:

1. Cut the mushroom in quarters after washing and pat drying. Add almond flour to a tray. Whisk eggs in a bowl. Add pork Panko to a separate plate along with garlic powder, onion powder, paprika, Italian seasoning, salt, and pepper.
2. Now toss mushrooms in almond flour. Then coat it with egg wash. Then cover it in pork rinds. Repeat for all the mushrooms.
3. Arrange the mushrooms in an air fryer basket lined with parchment paper. Air fry it for 7 minutes at 390 ° F (200°C). Serve it once done.

Per serving:

Calories 643 | Total Fat 39.7g 51% | Total Carbohydrate 10g 4% | Dietary Fiber 1g 4% | Protein 62.2g

— Pepperoni Chips —

Prep: 10 Minutes | Cook Time: 8 Minutes | Makes: 1 Serving

Ingredients:

- 20 slices pepperoni

Directions:

1. Layer the air fryer basket with parchment paper. Now add the pepperoni slices inside the air fryer basket.
2. Air fry it for about 8 minutes at 360 ° F (180°C) it should be crispy by then. Remove the chips and let them cool, and then serve with the cheese dip of your choice.

Per serving:

Calories 272 | Total Fat 24.2g 31% | Total Carbohydrate 0g 0% | Dietary Fiber 0g 0% | Protein 12.5g

— Poppers Peppers —

Prep: 14 Minutes | Cook Time: 15 Minutes | Makes: 2 Servings

Ingredients:

- 2 eggs
- 1 pound (450gr) fresh jalapenos, halved lengthwise and seeded
- 10 ounces (280gr) of cream cheese, softened
- 3/4 cup cheddar cheese, shredded
- 3/4 cup Monterey Jack cheese, shredded
- 4 bacon strips, cooked and crumbled
- ¼teaspoon garlic powder
- ¼teaspoon chili powder
- Salt, to taste
- ¼teaspoon smoked paprika
- ½ cup pork rinds, grated
- ½ cup of Sour cream

Directions:

1. Whisk eggs in a bowl. Use a separate bowl. Cut the peppers lengthwise and discard the seeds. For pork rinds (pork Panko).
2. Combine cream cheese, cheddar cheese, jack cheese, bacon, garlic, powder, chili powder, salt, and paprika in a third bowl. Spoon the prepared cheese mixture into the pepper.
3. Dip the peppers in egg wash and then in the pork rinds. Put it inside the air fryer basket lined with parchment paper. Air fries it for 15 minutes at 360 ° F (180°C). Once done, serve.

Per serving:

Calories 710 | Total Fat 60.8g 78% | Total Carbohydrate 11.7g 4% | Dietary Fiber 3.3g 12% | Protein 32.8g

Candied Pecans in the Air Fryer

Prep: 14 Minutes | Cook Time: 15 Minutes | Makes: 6 Servings

Ingredients:

- ½ cup stevia
- 1 tablespoon Cinnamon
- 1 egg
- 1 tablespoon Vanilla
- 1 pound (450gr) of pecans
- 2 teaspoons Water, Pinch of salt

Directions:

1. Take a bowl and add stevia, cinnamon, and salt, and mix well. Whisk eggs in a bowl and add vanilla and water. Whisk it until frothy. Add pecans to the egg mix, and then dust pecans with the cinnamon mixture.
2. Air fryer it at 300 ° F (150°C) for 15 minutes, stirring halfway. Let it cool once done, and then serve.

Per serving:

Calories 546 | Total Fat 54.7g 70% | Total Carbohydrate 12g 4% | Dietary Fiber 8.7g 31% | Protein 9.1g

— Cinnamon Nut Scrolls —

Prep: 15 Minutes | Cook Time: 18-22 Minutes | Makes: 2 Servings

Ingredients:

- 1-½ cups almond flour
- 2 teaspoons stevia
- 2 ounces (60gr) butter, cold
- ½ cup almond milk
- 1 egg
- ½ cup walnuts, chopped
- ½ cup slivered almonds, toasted
- 2 tablespoons stevia
- 1 teaspoon cinnamon, grounded

Directions:

1. Preheat the air fryer to around 390 ° F (200°C) and grease the basket with oil spray. Add almond flour and stevia in a bowl and mix with butter; whisk the egg with milk, and put it into the almond flour, incorporating dough. Knead it for 30 seconds and roll it in a rectangle. Mix the remaining ingredients in a bowl and top it over the dough.
2. Roll the dough into long strip-length. Cut-in pieces and roll to make a cinnamon bun style.
3. Put it in the air fryer basket and air fry it for 18-22 minutes at 400 ° F (205°C). Once done, serve.

Per serving:

Calories 413 | Total Fat 40.2g 51% | Total Carbohydrate 8.6g 3% | Dietary Fiber 4.6g 17% | Protein 10.7g

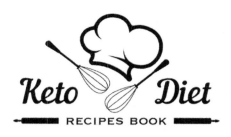

Chapter

7

Poultry Recipes

— Bacon Wrapped Thighs —

Prep: 22 Minutes | Cook Time: 22 Minutes | Makes: 3 Servings

Ingredients:

- 6 boneless, skinless chicken thighs
- Salt and black pepper, to taste
- 1 teaspoon of smoked paprika
- 16 tablespoons gruyere Swiss cheese, shredded
- 10-12 pieces large sliced bacon
- oil spray for greasing

Directions:

1. Preheat the air fryer before cooking at 380 ° F (195°C) for 5 minutes. Line a parchment paper onto the air fryer basket bottom.
2. Rub the chicken thighs with salt, black pepper, paprika, and Swiss cheese. Now wrap each thigh with a bacon strip, and use two strips if required. Make sure to cover the whole thigh with it.
3. Mist the thighs with oil spray and add them to an air fryer basket lined with parchment paper. Air fry it for 12 minutes at 370 ° F (190°C), flip the thighs and air fry for another 10 minutes; the internal meat thermometer reads 165 ° F (75°C) Once done, serve.

Per serving:

Calories 570 | Total Fat 37.5g 48% | Total Carbohydrate 0.4g 0% | Dietary Fiber 0.3g 1% | Protein 58.6g

— Chicken Bacon Poppers —

Prep: 15 Minutes | Cooking Time: 12 Minutes | Makes: 2 Servings

Ingredients:

- 1 pound (450gr) ground chicken
- 6 slices bacon, chopped
- ½ cup Mexican cheese
- ½ cup pork rinds, ground
- 1 egg, beaten
- 1 teaspoon minced garlic
- 1 teaspoon onion powder
- 1 teaspoon dill
- 1 teaspoon salt and black pepper

Directions:

1. Start by preheating the air fryer to around 400 ° F (205°C). Add all the listed ingredients in a bowl and mix them. From the mixture, make round balls.
2. Line the bottom of the basket with parchment paper and arrange the chicken balls on it. Air fryer for around 12 minutes at 400 ° F (205°C) until internal temperature reaches 165 ° F (75°C).. When done, take them out and serve.

Per serving:

Calories 791 | Total Fat 51.3g 66% | Total Carbohydrate 3.7g 1% | Dietary Fiber 0.5g 2% | Protein 78.4g

Montréal Chicken Breasts with Chipotle Sauce

Prep: 14 Minutes | Cook Time: 18-20 Minutes| Makes: 2 Servings

Chipotle Sauce ingredient:

- 6-ounce (170gr) chipotles in adobo sauce
- ½ cup sour cream
- 1/3 cup mayonnaise
- 2 tablespoons chopped cilantro
- ½ teaspoon cayenne powder
- 1 teaspoon garlic powder
- 1/3 teaspoon cumin
- Salt to taste

Chicken Ingredients:

- 4 large chicken breasts, 6 ounces (170gr) each
- 2 tablespoons Montreal chicken seasoning
- 1 teaspoon of thyme
- 1 teaspoon of cumin
- ¼teaspoon of paprika
- Oil spray for greasing, Salt, to taste

Directions:

1. Combine the entire chipotle sauce ingredient in a bowl and mix well. Set it aside. Next, rub the chicken with Montréal chicken seasoning thyme, cumin, paprika, and salt. Mist the chicken with oil spray.
2. Arrange the wings onto the basket of the air fryer. Air fry it at 390 ° F (200°C) for 18-20 minutes, flipping halfway. Once it's done, serve it with prepared sauce.

Per serving:

Calories 882 | Total Fat 50.6g 65% | Total Carbohydrate 16.7g 6% | Dietary Fiber 7.1g 25% |Protein 90.4g

Chicken Bites

Prep: 16 Minutes | Cooking Time: 12 Minutes | Makes: 2 Servings

Ingredients:

- 1 pound (450gr) chicken breast, cubes
- 2 tablespoons olive oil
- 1-½ teaspoons Cajun seasoning

Directions:

1. Start by preheating the air fryer to around 400 ° F (205°C). Coat the chicken with oil and toss it around in the seasoning.
2. Line the bottom of the basket of the air fryer with parchment paper. Then arrange the chicken, cooking it for around 12 minutes at about 350 ° F (180°C).. When done, serve it with the side of choice.

Per serving:

Calories 379 | Total Fat 19.7g 25% | Total Carbohydrate 0g 0% | Dietary Fiber 0g 0% | Protein 48.1g

Wings with Blue Cheese Dressing

Prep: 15 Minutes | Cook Time: 16 Minutes| Makes: 4 Servings

Ingredients:

- 6 tablespoons of butter
- Salt and black pepper, to taste
- 2 tablespoons of avocado oil
- 2 pounds (900gr) of chicken wings split at the joint
- Oil spray for greasing
- 1 cup blue cheese dressing

Directions:

1. Combine butter, salt, and pepper in a bowl and add avocado oil. Mix it well and coat the wings with it. Add the wings inside the air fryer basket lined with parchment paper.
2. Cook it for 16 minutes at 390 ° F (200°C), flipping halfway through. Once cooked, serve and enjoy with blue cheese dressing.

Per serving:

Calories 1130 | Total Fat 94.5g 121% | Total Carbohydrate 5g 2% | Dietary Fiber 0.3g 1% | Protein 64.1g

Crumbed Chicken Schnitzel

Prep: 10 Minutes | Cook Time: 16 Minutes| Makes: 4 Servings

Ingredients:

- 4 chicken fillets
- 1 cup pork rinds
- 1 teaspoon herb seasoning
- 2 eggs, lightly whisked
- 1/3 cup almond flour
- Salt and pepper, to taste

Directions:

1. Start by placing half the chicken between two plastic sheets and pound it using a pan or rolling pin. Do this with the other half and make the chicken as flat as possible.
2. Mix grated pork rinds and herb seasoning. In a small bowl, whisk the eggs. In a third bowl, add almond flour and mix it with salt and pepper.
3. Take the chicken pieces and coat them first with almond flour, then with eggs, and finally with pork rinds. Once covered, place it in the fridge for around 20 minutes.
4. Once rested, shift the chicken to the air fryer basket and cook it for around 16 minutes at about 400 ° F (205°C). When done, serve with the side of coleslaw.

Per serving:

Calories 492 | Total Fat 26.5g 34% | Total Carbohydrate 3.6g 1% | Dietary Fiber 1.8g 6% | Protein 59.3g

— Lemon Feta Chicken Breasts —

Prep: 10 Minutes | Cook Time: 20-22 Minutes| Makes: 1Serving

Ingredients:

- 2 boneless and skinless chicken breasts (8 ounces each(230gr))
- 4 tablespoons lemon juice
- 1 teaspoon dried oregano
- salt and black pepper, to taste
- 6 tablespoons crumbled feta cheese

Directions:

1. Preheat the air fryer before cooking at 400 ° F (205°C) for 4 minutes. Season the chicken breasts with lemon juice, dried oregano, salt, and black pepper. Add the chicken breast to an oil-greased baking dish.
2. Air fry it for 20-22 minutes at 400 ° F (205°C), flipping halfway through. When 5 minutes remain, top it with feta cheese. Once cooked, serve.

Per serving:

Calories 490 | Total Fat 20.7g 27% | Total Carbohydrate 5.5g 2% | Dietary Fiber 0.9g 3% | Protein 66.2g

Finger-Licking Chicken Fingers

Prep: 10Minutes | Cook Time: 16-20 Minutes| Makes: 2 Servings

Ingredients:

- 1 pound chicken breasts, boneless skinless (cut in to fingers)
- 1 cup almond milk
- Salt and black pepper, to taste
- 1 cup almond flour
- 2 tablespoons taco seasoning
- ½ cup coconut flour
- 1 cup sour cream, side serving

Directions:

1. Preheat the air fryer before cooking at 400 ° F (450gr) for 5 minutes. Use a meat mallet to pound the breast pieces. Then cut into finger shapes. Whisk the almond milk, salt, and black pepper in a bowl. Spread almond flour, taco seasoning, and coconut flour in a dish. Dip chicken in milk and then coat with flour. Arrange chicken in an air fryer basket lined with parchment paper. Air fry it for 16-20 minutes at 400 ° F (450gr), flipping halfway through. Serve with sour cream.

Per serving:

Calories 896 | Total Fat 52g 67% | Total Carbohydrate 25.8g 9% | Dietary Fiber 9g 32%| Protein 79.3g

— Chicken Wings —

Prep: 15 Minutes | Cook Time: 16 Minutes| Makes: 2 Servings

Ingredients:

- 2 teaspoons olive oil
- 2 teaspoons garlic salt
- 2 teaspoons lemon pepper
- 1/3 cup parmesan cheese, grated
- 1 pound (450gr) chicken wings split into flats

Directions:

1. Add olive oil, garlic salt, lemon pepper, and grated parmesan cheese. Mix it well and coat the wings with it. Toss the wings well and add to the air fryer basket lined with parchment paper.
2. Air fry it at 400 ° F (205°C) for 16 minutes, flipping halfway. Once it's crisp and golden brown, serve it with grated parmesan cheese.

Per serving:

Calories 918 | Total Fat 64g 82% |Total Carbohydrate 10.3g 4% | Dietary Fiber 1.1g4% | | Protein 73.4g

Spicy Chicken Breast with Green Beans

Prep: 20 Minutes | Cook Time: 22 Minutes| Makes: 2 Servings

Ingredients:

- 4 eggs, whisked
- 4 tablespoons of almond milk
- 1 cup of almond flour
- 2 tablespoons of Italian seasoning
- 1 teaspoon of paprika
- salt and black pepper, to taste
- 4 chicken breasts
- Oil spray for greasing
- 1 cup green beans
- 1 cup grated parmesan cheese, hard

Directions:

1. Whisk eggs in a bowl, add almond milk, and mix for good incorporation. Add almond flour, Italian season, paprika, salt, and pepper in a separate bowl. Coat the green beans and chicken with flour spice rub.
2. Then arrange both side by side on the air fryer basket lined with parchment paper. Air fry it for 22 minutes at 390 ° F (200°C).
3. Take out the green beans after 12 minutes and cook the chicken. Flip the breast piece halfway through. Once done, serve with grated parmesan cheese on top.

Per serving:

Calories 1165 | Total Fat 67.2g 86% | Total Carbohydrate 14.4g 5% | Dietary Fiber 4.4g 16% | Protein 127.5g

Hot Buffalo wings with Blue Cheese Dressing

Prep: 15 Minutes | Cook Time: 12 Minutes | Makes: 4 Servings

Ingredients:

- 4 tablespoons of butter
- 2 teaspoons of olive oil
- Salt and black pepper, to taste
- 1 cup hot sauce
- 2 pounds (900gr) of chicken wings split at the joint
- Oil spray for greasing
- 1 cup blue cheese dressing for serving

Directions:

1. Mix butter with oil, salt, pepper, and hot sauce. Add the wings to the mixture and toss it around to coat evenly. Line the bottom of the air fryer with parchment paper.
2. Once coated, arrange them in the greased air fryer basket with oil spray, and cook them for around 12 minutes at 370 ° F (190°C). When done, shift them to a serving plate and serve them with blue cheese.

Per serving:

Calories 1166 | Total Fat 96.5g 124% | Total Carbohydrate 11g 4% | Dietary Fiber 0.4g 1% | Protein 62.6g

— Turkey Patties —

Prep: 16 Minutes | Cook Time: 6-8 Minutes | Makes: 3 Servings

Ingredients:

- 3 ounces (85gr) almond flour, grounded
- 1.5 pounds (680gr) lean turkey, grounded
- 1 cup feta cheese, crumbled
- Salt and black pepper, to taste
- ½ cup tomatoes, chopped
- 2 red onions, chopped
- Oil spray for greasing

Directions:

1. Start by adding almond flour, ground turkey, cheese, salt, pepper, tomatoes, and onions in a bowl and mixing them thoroughly. Take a small portion from the mixture and shape them into patties.
2. Spray oil on both sides of the patties and arrange them in the air fryer basket greased with oil spray, cooking them for around 6-8 minutes on each side at 400 ° F (205°C). When done, place them and serve warm.

Per serving:

Calories 714 | Total Fat 36.3g 47% | Total Carbohydrate 16.1g 6% | Dietary Fiber 5g 18% | Protein 80.6g

— Cheesy Chicken Sausages —

Prep: 12 Minutes | Cook Time: 16 Minutes | Makes: 4 Servings

Ingredients:

- 4 cups chicken, minced
- 2 small carrots, peeled and grated
- 1 cup zucchini, peeled and grated
- ½ cup cheddar cheese
- ½ cup pork rinds
- 1 green onion, chopped
- 2 teaspoons of Vegemite Squeeze
- 2 garlic cloves, crushed
- 1 egg, lightly beaten
- Oil spray for greasing, Salt and black pepper.
- Hot sauce, as per liking

Directions:

1. Add minced chicken, carrots, zucchini, cheese, and pork rinds in a bowl. Then add green onions, vegemite, and garlic and remix it. Season accordingly with salt and pepper and remix it. Add one egg and combine all the ingredients.
2. Make sausages by hand and grease the links with oil spray.
3. Arrange the sausages in an air fryer basket lined with parchment paper. Air fry it for 16 minutes at 370 ° F (190°C), flipping halfway through. When done, serve it with a side of hot sauce.

Per serving:

Calories 286 | Total Fat 13.5g 17% | Total Carbohydrate 4.5g 2% | Dietary Fiber 1.1g 4% | Protein 35.8g

— Lemon Feta Chicken —

Prep: 25 Minutes | Cook Time: 16-20 Minutes | Makes: 2 Servings

Ingredients:

- 2 chicken breasts, skinless, halved
- 1 tablespoon lemon juice
- Salt and black pepper, to taste
- ½ teaspoon oregano, dried
- 2 tablespoons feta cheese, crumbled

Directions:

1. Start by preheating the air fryer to 400 ° F (205°C).. Drizzle some oil in a pan and arrange the chicken breasts in them. Add lemon juice over them and season them with salt, pepper, oregano, and feta cheese. Then shift the pan to the air fryer, cooking it for at least 16-20 minutes. Once the chicken reaches an internal temperature of 165 ° F (75°C), take it out and serve.

Per serving:

Calories 100 | Total Fat 3.5g 5% | Total Carbohydrate 0.8g 0% | Dietary Fiber 0.2g 1% | Protein 15.2g

— Pistachio Crusted Chicken —

Prep: 12 Minutes | Cook Time: 18-20 Minutes| Makes: 2 Servings

Ingredients:

- 2(6 ounces each(170gr)) chicken breast, boneless, skinless
- 4 tablespoons of mayonnaise
- Salt and black pepper, to taste, Oil spray
- ½ cup roasted pistachios, crushed

Directions:

1. Start by washing and then patting the chicken using a kitchen towel. Then coat it evenly with mayo and season with salt and pepper. Coat it with grated pistachios. Then, arrange the chicken in the air fryer and lightly coat it with oil.
2. Cook it for around 18-20 minutes at about 370 ° F (190°C). Make sure to flip it halfway to ensure even cooking. When done, serve.

Per serving:

Calories 1065 | Total Fat 41.6g 53% | Total Carbohydrate 15.6g 6% | Dietary Fiber 3.3g 12% | Protein 149.6g

— Fajita-Stuffed Chicken —

Prep: 15 Minutes | Cook Time: 16 Minutes| Makes: 3 Servings

Ingredients:

- 4 small onions, halved and thinly sliced
- 1 medium green pepper, thinly sliced
- 12 ounces (340gr) cheddar cheese, sliced
- ½ teaspoon garlic powder
- Salt and black pepper, to taste
- 1 teaspoon ground cumin
- 4 tablespoons olive oil
- 2 tablespoons chili powder
- 6 boneless and skinless chicken breasts

Side serving:

- Sour cream, as needed
- Jalapeno slices, as needed

Directions:

1. First, preheat the appliance to 390 ° F (200°C) before starting the cooking for 6 minutes. Add onion, green pepper, cheddar cheese, garlic powder, salt, pepper, cumin, and olive oil.
2. Then butterfly cut the chicken breasts. Fill the cavity with this prepared mixture.
3. Place chicken onto an air-fryer basket lined with parchment paper. Air fry it for 16 minutes at 400 ° F (205°C). Flip the chicken halfway through. Serve with listed toppings.

Per serving:

Calories 1211 | Total Fat 79.5g 102% | Total Carbohydrate 18.1g 7% | Dietary Fiber 4.5g16% | Protein 105.6g

— Boneless Chicken —

Prep: 12 Minutes | Cook Time: 10-12 Minutes| Makes: 2 Servings

Ingredients:

- chicken breasts, frozen boneless, skinless (8 ounces each(230gr))
- 3 tablespoons avocado oil
- Salt and black pepper, to taste
- 1 cup of unsweetened barbecue sauce

Directions:

1. Start by preheating the air fryer to around 400 ° F (205°C). Coat the chicken with avocado oil and then season it with salt and pepper.
2. Grease the inside of the air fryer with oil and place the breast in the basket, cooking it for around 10-12 minutes and flipping it halfway through the cooking process at 400 ° F (205°C). Baste the chicken breast with bbq every 3 minutes. When done, shift it to a serving plate and serve.

Per serving:

Calories 583 | Total Fat 24.3g 31% | Total Carbohydrate 1.2g 0% | Dietary Fiber 0.9g 3% | Protein 84.8g

— Hot Parmesan Chicken Wings —

Prep: 15Minutes | Cook Time: 16-18 Minutes| Makes: 4 Servings

Sauce Ingredients:

- ¼cup stevia
- 1 tablespoon hot sauce
- ¼ cup coconut amino
- 4 teaspoons of sesame oil
- 1/3 teaspoon of red pepper flakes
- Salt and black pepper, to taste

Ingredients for chicken:

- 8 chicken wings
- ½ cup parmesan cheese, hard and grated

Directions:

1. Put all the sauce ingredients in a large bowl and whisk it well. Now coat the wings with the sauce and add it to the air fryer basket lined with parchment paper.
2. Air fry it at 390 ° F (200°C) for 16-18 minutes, flipping halfway through. Baste the chicken with leftover sauce every 5 minutes. Once cooked, serve and enjoy with grated parmesan cheese on top.

Per serving:

Calories 955 | Total Fat 65.9g 84% | Total Carbohydrate 0.9g 0% | Dietary Fiber 0.1g 0% | Protein 85.2g

— Classic Chicken Thighs —

Prep: 14 Minutes | Cook Time: 18-22 Minutes | Makes: 2 Servings

Ingredients:

- 4 tablespoons of the peach preserve (sugar-free)
- Salt and black pepper, to taste
- 2 tablespoons Lemon Juice
- 6 -8 chicken thighs bone-in
- Oil spray for greasing

Directions:

1. Start by mixing peach preserves, salt, black pepper, and lemon juice in a large bowl. Once properly mixed, add the chicken thighs to the bowl and toss them around until they are wholly coated. Let it sit for 30 minutes to marinate.
2. Grease the basket of the air fryer with oil spray. Next, arrange the thighs in the basket. Cook chicken in the air fryer for around 18-22 minutes at 400 ° F (205°C), and flip them halfway through the cooking.
3. When done, serve the thighs with your favorite keto-based sauce.

Per serving:

Calories 935 | Total Fat 32.7g 42% | Total Carbohydrate 26g 9% | Dietary Fiber 0g 0% | Protein 126.7g

— Perfect Chicken —

Prep: 10 Minutes | Cook Time: 18-20 Minutes | Makes: 2 Servings

Ingredients:

- ½ tablespoon lemon juice
- 1 teaspoon chicken seasoning
- Salt and black pepper, to taste
- ½ teaspoon of garlic powder
- 2 chicken breasts, halved
- Oil spray for greasing
- ½ cup provolone cheese
- ½ cup blue cheese, crumbled

Directions:

1. Start by adding lemon juice to a bowl and mixing it with chicken seasoning, salt, pepper, and garlic powder. Add the chicken breasts to the bowl and coat the chicken with the seasoning.
2. Grease the basket of air fryer with oil and arrange the chicken, cooking for around 18-20 minutes at about 350 ° F (180°C)..
3. While the chicken is cooking, add blue cheese, and provolone cheese in a saucepan and let it cook until all combined into a sauce consistency. Once the chicken is done, serve it with a cheese sauce.

Per serving:

Calories 518 | Total Fat 29.6g 38% | Total Carbohydrate 2.1g 1% | Dietary Fiber 0.1g 0% | Protein 58.1g

— Chicken Breast —

Prep: 25 Minutes | Cook Time: 10-15 Minutes | Makes: 2 Servings

Ingredients:

- 4 boneless chicken breasts
- 2 tablespoons butter
- ¼ teaspoon garlic powder
- ½ teaspoon salt
- ¼ teaspoon pepper

Directions:

1. Start by preheating the air fryer to around 390 ° F (200°C).. Arrange the breasts on a cutting board. Place butter in the microwave and heat it till melted, then add garlic powder, salt, and pepper to the butter and mix it. Add the butter mix and coat them evenly with it.
2. Once coated, shift them into the air fryer basket and cook them for around 10 to 15 minutes at 380 ° F (195°C). Cook the chicken until it reaches 165 ° F (75°C) internal, and flip it halfway through the cooking. When done, take it out and serve or place it in the fridge to enjoy later.

Per serving:

Calories 658 | Total Fat 33.2g 43% | Total Carbohydrate 0.4g 0% | Dietary Fiber 0.1g 0% | Protein 84.7g

— Cosmic Wings —

Prep: 10 Minutes | Cook Time: 12 Minutes | Makes: 4 Servings

Ingredients:

- 1 tablespoon garlic powder
- ½ tablespoon onion powder
- ½ tablespoon paprika
- 1 tablespoon dried parsley
- 1 /3 teaspoon of rosemary
- ¼ teaspoon salt, oil spray for greasing
- ¼teaspoon pepper
- 1.5 pounds (680gr) of chicken wings
- 6 ounces (170gr) of Cosmic Sauce

Directions:

1. Start by mixing garlic powder, onion powder, paprika, parsley, rosemary, salt, and pepper in a bowl. Put the chicken into the bowl and toss it around to coat evenly.
2. Grease the bottom of the air fryer with oil and arrange the chicken in it, cooking it for around 12 minutes at about 375 ° F (190°C), making sure to flip it halfway. When done, toss it with cosmic jerry sauce and serve.

Per serving:

Calories 338 | Total Fat 12.9g 17% | Total Carbohydrate 2.9g 1% | Dietary Fiber 0.7g 2% | Protein 49.8g

Pickle Mayo Chicken Tenders

Prep: 15 Minutes | Cook Time: 6 Minutes | Makes: 4 Servings

Ingredients:

- 2 pounds (900gr) of chicken tenderloins
- 2 tablespoons of poultry seasoning
- 2 teaspoons of olive oil
- Oil spray for greasing
- 1 cup mayonnaise
- 2 teaspoons of pickled ginger, reserved 2 tsp pickling liquid

Directions:

1. Start by seasoning the chicken with poultry seasoning and olive oil. Grease the basket with oil spray and arrange the chicken.
2. Put the basket inside the air fryer and cook it for around 6 minutes at about 400 ° F (205°C), flipping halfway through.
3. While the chicken is cooking, mix mayo and pickle liquid in a bowl. Once the chicken is cooked, serve it with the mayo sauce.

Per serving:

Calories 324 | Total Fat 25.1g 32% | Total Carbohydrate 16.4g 6% | Dietary Fiber 0.3g 1% | Protein 9.8g

Chicken with Blue Cheese

Prep: 20 Minutes | Cook Time: 18-20 Minutes | Makes: 2 Servings

Ingredients:

- 4 chicken breasts, halved
- 2 tablespoons lemon juice
- 2 tablespoons of Chayote squash juice
- Salt and black pepper, to taste
- 2 teaspoons chicken seasoning
- ¼ cup blue cheese, crumbled

Directions:

1. Start by preheating the air fryer to around 400 ° F (205°C) for at least five minutes before cooking. Add the chicken, lemon juice, Chayote squash juice, salt, pepper, and chicken seasoning in a bowl. Mix everything and coat the chicken evenly throughout.
2. Once coated, arrange the chicken in the basket. Air fry at 370 ° F (190°C) for 16-18 minutes.
3. Make sure to flip it halfway to ensure even cooking throughout. Take the chicken out and serve it with blue cheese.

Per serving:

Calories 622 | Total Fat 26.6g 34% | Total Carbohydrate 1.6g 1% | Dietary Fiber 0.2g 1% | Protein 88.4g

Savory Chicken Breast

Prep: 15 Minutes | Cook Time: 20 Minutes | Makes: 4 Servings

Ingredients:

- 4 chicken breasts
- ½ cup olive oil
- 2 tablespoons soy sauce
- 2 tablespoons balsamic vinegar
- 1/3 cup brown sugar
- ½ tablespoon of garlic powder
- 1 teaspoon of onion powder
- salt & pepper to taste

Directions:

1. Start by preheating the air fryer to around 400 ° F (205°C). Mix all the listed ingredients in a bowl and mix them. Cover the chicken entirely and let it sit in the marinade for at least a few hours.
2. Grease the basket of the chicken with oil spray, poke it with a fork, and place it in the air fryer basket, cooking it for around 16-18 minutes at 370 ° F (190°C). Make sure to flip the chicken halfway in the cooking to ensure an even cook throughout. Once the internal temperature of the chicken reaches around 165 ° F (75°C), take it out of the basket and serve.

Per serving:

Calories 553 | Total Fat 36g 46% | Total Carbohydrate 13.9g 5% | Dietary Fiber 0.2g 1% | Protein 43.4g

Easy Turkey Meatballs

Prep: 16 Minutes | Cook Time: 10-14 Minutes | Makes: 2 Servings

Ingredients:

- 1 pound (450gr) of ground turkey
- ½ cup pork rinds, grated
- 1 egg
- salt and black pepper, to taste
- ¼cup fresh parsley
- 1 tablespoon low-sodium soy sauce
- Oil spray for greasing

Directions:

1. Mix turkey with pork rinds, eggs, salt, pepper, parsley, and soy sauce. Take small portions of the mix and shape them into balls. Arrange them in the air fryer basket and spray some oil on them.
2. Cook them for around 10-14 minutes at about 350 ° F (180°C). Make sure to flip the meatballs halfway in the cooking to ensure they even cook throughout. When done, serve and enjoy.

Per serving:

Calories 602 | Total Fat 34.9g 45% | Total Carbohydrate 1.2g 0% | Dietary Fiber 0.3g 1% | Protein 79.1g

— Chicken Tomatina —

Prep: 16 Minutes | Cook Time: 18-20 Minutes| Makes: 4 Servings

Ingredients:

- 1 teaspoon of ginger garlic paste
- ¼ cup fresh basil leaves
- 2 tablespoons olive oil
- Salt and black pepper, to taste
- 3/4 cup lemon juice
- 2 plum tomatoes
- 4 chicken breasts, boneless and skinless

Directions:

1. Start by blending ginger, garlic paste, basil, oil, salt, pepper, and lemon juice in the blender until they form a paste. Then add in the tomatoes and pulse it in to smooth paste.
2. Place the tomato paste in the refrigerator and let it rest for at least 40 minutes so that the flavors develop nicely.
3. Place an oil-greased round pan in the air fryer basket and place the chicken in it, pouring the sauce over it.
4. Cook it for 18 to 20 minutes at 370 ° F (190°C), flipping halfway through. When it's done, serve the chicken.

Per serving:

Calories 405 | Total Fat 18.7g 24% |Total Carbohydrate 13.6g 5% | Dietary Fiber 2.9g 10% | Protein 45.6g

Sesame Chicken Breast with Veggies and Feta Salad

Prep: 25 Minutes | Cook Time: 18-22 Minutes| Makes: 4 Servings

Ingredients:

- 4 tablespoons of sesame oil
- 2 tablespoons of sesame seeds
- 2 tablespoons of stevia
- 2 tablespoons coconut amino
- Salt and black pepper, pinch
- 2 tablespoons of lemon juice
- 2 pounds (900gr) of chicken breasts

Salad Ingredients:

- ¼ cup sour cream
- 2 tablespoons white wine vinegar
- 2 teaspoons dill weed, chopped
- 1 large English cucumber, cut crosswise into 1/3-inch slices (8mm)
- 1 large red onion, sliced
- 1 red tomato, chopped
- 1 cup arugula, roughly chopped
- Salt and black pepper, to taste
- 1 cup feta cheese, salt and black pepper, to taste

Directions:

1. Mix sesame oil, sesame seeds, stevia, coconut aminos, salt pepper, lemon juice, and chicken. Let the chicken rest and then marinate for at least 30 minutes.
2. Preheat the air fryer to around 400 ° F (205°C) and add the chicken to the basket once the air fryer is preheated for 2 minutes. Cook the chicken for about 18-20 minutes at 400 ° F (205°C), and flip it halfway while cooking.
3. Meanwhile, add all the ingredients for the salad in a bowl and mix them. Once the chicken is done cooking, serve it with the side of the salad.

Per serving:

Calories 727 | Total Fat 43.8g 56% | Total Carbohydrate 7.6g 3% | Dietary Fiber 1.6g 6% | Protein 72.9g

— Classic Chicken Nuggets —

Prep: 15 Minutes | Cook Time: 18-20 Minutes| Makes: 4 Servings

Ingredients:

- 1 cup pickle juice
- 2 pounds (900gr) of chicken breasts cut into cubes

Breading Ingredients:

- 1 cup almond flour
- 2 teaspoons cayenne pepper
- 1 teaspoon of stevia
- ¼ teaspoon paprika
- ¼ teaspoon chili powder
- Salt and black pepper, to taste
- ½ teaspoon baking soda

Other Ingredients:

- 1 cup coconut milk
- 2 large eggs

Directions:

1. Start by adding pickle juice to a bowl and marinating the chicken for at least 10 minutes. While the chicken is marinating, mix breading ingredients, including almond flour, cayenne pepper, stevia, paprika, chili powder, salt, pepper, and baking soda.
2. In a separate large bowl, whisk eggs with the coconut milk. Once the chicken is marinated for enough time, take it out and coat it first with eggs and then with flour.
3. Shake the extra flour and arrange them in a heated air fryer at around 370 ° F (190°C). Cook it for about 18-20 minutes at 370 ° F (190°C), and flip them halfway through the cooking. When done, serve.

Per serving:

Calories 635 | Total Fat 36 g 46% | Total Carbohydrate 6.4g 2% | Dietary Fiber 2.8 g 10% | Protein 70g

— Zesty and Spiced Chicken —

Prep: 22 Minutes | Cook Time: 18-25 Minutes| Makes: 3Servings

Ingredients:

- 2 cloves of garlic, minced
- 1-inch (25mm) ginger paste
- 1-½ tablespoons of lemon juice
- ¼ teaspoon of lemon zest
- 2 tablespoons olive oil
- 2 cups plain yogurt
- Salt and black pepper, to taste
- 1 teaspoon of red chili powder
- 1 teaspoon of turmeric powder
- 1 teaspoon of thyme
- 1 teaspoon of five-spice powder
- 1.5 pounds (680gr) chicken breasts, boneless and skinless

Directions:

1. Start by adding all the listed ingredients in a bowl and mixing them. Add the chicken to the bowl and toss it around, evenly coating the slides. Place the marinated chicken in the fridge for at least 2 hours.
2. Once the chicken is well rested, grease the air fryer basket with oil and add it to it, cooking it for around 18 to 25 minutes at 400 ° F (205°C), when done, take it out and serve.

Per serving:

Calories 478 | Total Fat 21.3g 27% | Total Carbohydrate 10.1g 4% | Dietary Fiber 0.5g 2% |Protein 56.5g

Glazed Tomato — Chicken Kabobs —

Prep: 35Minutes | Cook Time: 22 Minutes| Makes: 3Servings

Glazed Ingredients:

- ¼cup stevia
- ½ cup coconut amino
- ½ cup lime juice
- 1 teaspoon of garlic powder

Chicken Ingredients:

- 4 garlic cloves, minced
- Salt and black pepper, to taste
- 1 tablespoon oregano
- 1 cup Greek yogurt, plain
- ½ teaspoon lemon zest
- 2 lemon juice, Salt and black pepper, to taste
- ¼ cup extra-virgin olive oil
- 1.5-pounds (680gr) chicken breast, boneless, skinless, and cut into cubes of 2 inches

- 2 large red tomatoes, quarter
- 2 large red onions, quartered

Directions:

1. Start by mixing the glaze ingredients in a bowl and mixing them correctly. In another bowl, add garlic, salt, pepper, oregano, yogurt, lemon zest, and Juice, and oil; mix them. Then add the chicken to the mixture and coat it evenly on all sides.
2. Let it rest for at least one hour at room temperature before cooking them.
3. Take a skewer long enough for the air fryer basket and skewer tomato, chicken, and onions alternating. Once skewered, arrange them in the air fryer and fry them for around 18-22 minutes at 400 ° F (205°C). When done, take them out, glaze them with the glaze made earlier, and serve.

Per serving:

Calories 618 | Total Fat 24.3g 31% | Total Carbohydrate 25.8g 9% | Dietary Fiber 3g 11% | Protein 73.1g

— Zesty Chicken Breasts —

Prep: 10 Minutes | Cook Time: 22 Minutes | Makes: 4 Servings

Ingredients:

- 4 boneless skinless chicken breasts (8 ounces each (230gr))
- 2 tablespoons arrowroot powder
- Salt and black pepper, to taste, Oil spray

Ingredients for Lemon Sauce:

- ½ cup lemon juice
- 3 tablespoons stevia
- 1 tablespoon coconut amino
- 1 tablespoon lemon juice
- 1 teaspoon of orange zest
- ½ teaspoon of ginger
- 2 teaspoons Xanthan Gum+2 teaspoons water

Directions:

1. Preheat the air fryer before cooking at 400 ° F (205°C) for a few minutes. Coat the chicken with arrowroot powder, salt, and pepper.
2. Mist it with oil spray and add it to the air fryer basket lined with parchment paper. Air fry it for 22 minutes at 400 ° F (205°C), flipping halfway through.
3. Meanwhile, whisk the entire lemon sauce ingredient in a bowl and add it to the saucepan. Simmer it down to the thickest. Once the chicken is ready, add it to the saucepan, and coat it well. Serve and enjoy.

Per serving:

Calories 223 | Total Fat 4.6g 6% | Total Carbohydrate 0.3g 0% | Dietary Fiber 0.1g 0% | Protein 42.3g

Parmesan Chicken Tenders

Prep: 10 Minutes | Cook Time: 12 Minutes| Makes: 2 Servings

Ingredients:

- 2 eggs
- ½ cup coconut milk
- 1 cup parmesan cheese, grated
- ½ cup pork rinds
- ¼ teaspoon of paprika
- Salt and pepper, to taste
- 1 pound (450gr) skinless chicken breast, cut into strips
- 2 teaspoons of avocado oil

Directions:

1. Whisk eggs together with coconut milk. Mix parmesan cheese, pork rinds, paprika, salt, and pepper in another bowl. Start by coating the chicken first with eggs and then adding them to the pork rinds mixture.
2. Place the chicken in the air fryer basket and drizzle some oil, cooking it for around 12 minutes at about 400 ° F (205°C). When it's done, serve.

Per serving:

Calories 1029 | Total Fat 61.6g 79% | Total Carbohydrate 7.1g 3% | Dietary Fiber 1.6g 6% | Protein 113.1g

Nashville Hot Chicken

Prep: 20 Minutes | Cook Time: 12 Minutes| Makes: 4 Servings

Ingredients:

- 2 tablespoons dill pickle juice, divided
- 2 tablespoons hot pepper sauce, divided
- Salt and black pepper, to taste
- 2 pounds (900gr) of chicken tenders
- 1 cup almond flour
- 2 large eggs
- 1 cup cream
- 1 tablespoon cayenne pepper
- 2 tablespoons stevia
- ½ teaspoon paprika
- 1 teaspoon chili powder
- ½ teaspoon garlic powder
- ½ cup olive oil
- Salt and black pepper, to taste
- Few Dill pickle slices

Directions:

1. Start by mixing 1 tablespoon pickle juice with 1 tablespoon hot sauce and seasoning of salt and black pepper. Add the chicken and toss it around to coat the chicken tenders evenly. Place it in the fridge for about 2 hours to let the taste properly develops.

2. Add almond flour, salt, and black pepper in a bowl. In another bowl, crack the eggs with cream, remaining pickle juice, and hot sauce.
3. Take the marinated chicken and coat it with almond flour, dip it in the whisked eggs, then cover it again with almond flour.
4. Grease the bottom of the air fryer with oil and arrange the chicken on it. Cook the chicken for around 6 minutes on each side at about 375 ° F (190°C). While cooking, take a bowl and mix cayenne pepper, stevia, paprika, chili powder, garlic powder, oil, salt, and freshly ground black pepper. Once the chicken is done, toss it in the seasoning mixture and serve with pickled slices.

Per serving:

Calories 770 | Total Fat 51.7g 66% |Total Carbohydrate 5.1g 2% | Dietary Fiber 1.5g 5% | Protein 71.1g

Crispy Fillets with Sriracha Honey Sauce

Prep: 12 Minutes | Cook Time: 16 Minutes| Makes: 4 Servings

Chicken Batter Ingredients:

- ½ cup coconut milk
- ½ cup almond flour more if needed
- ½ cup arrowroot powder
- 2 eggs, whisked
- 2 teaspoons Sriracha sauce or to taste
- Salt and black pepper to taste

Sauce Ingredients:

- ½ cup mayonnaise
- 2 tablespoons stevia
- 2 tablespoons Sriracha sauce, to taste

Other Ingredients:

- 1 pound (450gr) of chicken breast cut in half
- 2 cups pork rinds, grated
- Oil spray for greasing

Directions:

1. Start by mixing all the ingredients for the batter in a bowl. In another bowl, add and mix all the ingredients for the sauce. Add pork rinds to a baking tray. Dip the chicken in the flour batter and coat it with pork rinds.
2. Grease the basket of the air fryer with oil and arrange the chicken in the basket, cooking it for around 16-18 minutes at about 350 ° F (180°C, making sure to flip them halfway through the cooking. When done, serve with prepared sauce.

Per serving:

Calories 552 | Total Fat 32.3g 41% | Total Carbohydrate 9.4g 3% | Dietary Fiber 0.4g 1% | Protein 55.8g

— Chicken Tenders —

Prep: 25 Minutes | Cook Time: 14 Minutes| Makes: 2 Servings

Ingredients:

- 2 eggs, whisked
- ½ cup powdered parmesan cheese, grated
- ½ cup almond flour
- Salt and black pepper, to taste
- 1 teaspoon cayenne pepper
- Oil spray for greasing
- 1.5 pounds (680gr) of chicken tenderloins

Directions:

1. Crack and beat the eggs in a small bowl. Add cheese, almond flour, salt, pepper, and cayenne pepper in a zip-lock bag and mix them. Grease the inside of the air fryer with oil. Dip the chicken tenders in the eggs and arrange them on another plate. Then add each tender to the zip lock bag and shake them to coat the chicken evenly.
2. Do this with all the tenders and arrange them in the air fryer basket, cooking them for around 12 minutes at 370 ° F (190°C). then increase the heat and cook them for 2 minutes at 400 ° F (205°C). When done, take them out and serve them with the dip of choice.

Per serving:

Calories 476 | Total Fat 31.6g 40% | Total Carbohydrate 9.6g 4% | Dietary Fiber 3.3g 12% | Protein 43.2g

Delicious Chicken Sausage Mix

Prep:15 Minutes | Cooking Time:40-45 Minutes | Makes: 4 Servings

Ingredients:

- 2 tablespoons olive oil
- 3 cloves minced garlic
- 1 diced onion
- 1 diced red bell pepper
- 1 diced green bell pepper
- 6 chicken sausage
- ⅓ cup butter
- ⅓ cup almond flour
- 3 cups chicken broth
- 1 cup diced celery
- 1 cup sliced okra
- 1 cup tomatoes, diced
- 1 pound (450gr) chicken breasts
- 2 bay leaves
- 2 teaspoons Creole seasoning
- salt and black pepper, to taste

Directions:

1. Start by adding oil, garlic, onions, bell peppers, and sausages in a bowl and tossing them. Line the bottom of the basket of the air fryer with parchment paper.
2. Shift the sausage mix to the basket of the unit and cook it for around 8 minutes at about 400 ° F(205°C).
3. Meanwhile, mix butter and almond flour in a pot while heating for 5 minutes. After five minutes, turn off the heat, pour the chicken broth, and mix the vegetables, diced tomatoes, chicken breast pieces, and bay leaves. Season it with Creole seasoning, salt, and black pepper. Give it a mix and cook it for around 20 minutes at 350 ° F (180°C).
4. When done, shift it to a serving plate and serve it with air fryer items.

Per serving:

Calories 689 | Total Fat 40.6g 52% | Total Carbohydrate 23.3g 8% | Dietary Fiber 4g 14% | Protein 57.9g

— Tandoori Chicken Thighs —

Prep: 15 Minutes | Cook Time: 18-22 Minutes| Makes: 4 Servings

Ingredients:

- 2 pounds (900gr) of chicken thighs or legs
- 1-½ cup plain yogurt
- 2-inches (50mm) ginger, crushed
- garlic cloves, crushed
- 1 teaspoon of red chili powder
- 1 tablespoon tandoori paste or powder
- ½ teaspoon turmeric
- ½ teaspoon coriander powder
- ½ teaspoon cumin powder
- 1 teaspoon Garam Masala
- Salt and black pepper, to taste
- 2 tablespoons lemon juice
- 2 tablespoons of clarified butter

Directions:

1. Start by adding and mixing all the ingredients in a bowl. Add the chicken to the bowl and coat them evenly throughout. Put the chicken in the refrigerator for 30 minutes and let it rest.
2. Preheat the air fryer before cooking for 6 minutes at 400 ° F (205°C). Take the chicken thighs and arrange them inside the basket of the air fryer lined with parchment paper, air frying at around 400 ° F (205°C) for about 18-22 minutes.
3. Make sure to flip the thighs halfway in the cooking to allow an even cook throughout. When done, remove it and serve.

Per serving:

Calories 678 | Total Fat 45.3g 58% | Total Carbohydrate 6.7g 2% | Dietary Fiber 0.4g 1% | Protein 56.8g

Crispy Chicken Fingers with Ranch Dressing

Prep: 15 Minutes | Cook Time: 12 Minutes | Makes: 4 Servings

Ingredients:

- 2 pounds (900gr) of chicken breast fillet, striped
- tablespoons olive oil
- salt, to taste
- 2 ounces (60gr) of ranch salad dressing & seasoning mix, gluten-free, keto
- 2 eggs, whisked
- 2 cups pork Panko or grated pork rinds

Directions:

1. Start by drizzling olive oil over the chicken and seasoning it with salt and ranch dressing. Whisk the eggs inside a large bowl. Add grated pork rinds in another bowl. Dip the marinated chicken first in eggs and then coat it with crumbs
2. Arrange the chicken in the air fryer, cooking it for around 12 minutes at about 400 ° F (205°C). make sure to flip the chicken halfway in the cooking to ensure an even cooking throughout. When done, serve the chicken with the desired seasoning.

Per serving:

Calories 822 | Total Fat 48g 62% | Total Carbohydrate 0.2g 0% | Dietary Fiber 0g 0% | Protein 95.4g

Chicken Kabobs with Onions and Bell Peppers

Prep: 20 Minutes | Cook Time: 16 Minutes | Makes: 4 Servings

Ingredients marinade:

- ½ cup red wine vinegar
- 1/3 cup olive oil
- 2 teaspoons dried oregano
- 4 minced garlic cloves
- 2 tablespoons finely chopped parsley
- salt and black pepper, to taste

Ingredients chicken kabobs:

- 2 pounds (900gr) chopped chicken breasts
- 2 sweet bell peppers, thick cubed
- 1 chopped onion, wedged cut
- 8 ounces (230gr) mushrooms

Toppings:

- Additional parsley chopped for garnishing

Directions:

1. Start by mixing all the ingredients for the marinade in a bowl. Once mixed, add the chicken and mix it till evenly coated throughout. Once covered, shift the bowl to the fridge and let it rest for at least 1 hour.
2. Soak the skewers, if using wooden ones, to prevent burning. Once the chicken has marinated, take the chicken out and thread it onto wooden skewers alternating between bell peppers, onions, and mushrooms
3. Preheat the air fryer to around 370 ° F (190°C) for 5 minutes and then arrange the skewers in the basket lined with parchment paper, cooking it for about 16 minutes at 370 °F (190°C). When done, serve with the garnish of parsley.

Per serving:

Calories 612 | Total Fat 33.9g 43% | Total Carbohydrate 6.3g 2% | Dietary Fiber 1.6g 6% | Protein 68g

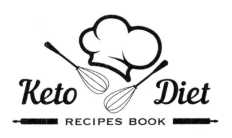

Chapter

8

Beef, Pork and Lamb

— Pork Bacon Wraps —

Prep: 15 Minutes | Cook Time: 15-18 Minutes| Makes: 2 Servings

Ingredients:

- 6 pork bacon, large slices
- 4 organic eggs, whisked
- 1 tablespoon chives, fresh and chopped
- 4 ounces (115gr) of cream cheese
- 4 -6 coconuts wraps
- Oil spray for greasing

Directions:

1. Start by preheating the air fryer to around 400 ° F (205°C) for 5 minutes before cooking. Cook the bacon in a large skillet till it is nice and crispy. Once cooked, take it off the pan and turn it into a crumble once it is cool enough.
2. In the same skillet, cook the eggs. Let it get cool.
3. Shift the egg to a bowl and mix it with bacon crumbs, chives, and cream cheese. Place a coconut wrap on a clean flat surface and roll it flat. Add the mixture to the center. Brush the edges with water and roll.
4. Place it in the air fryer basket and cook it for around 6 minutes at 350 ° F (180°C), making sure to flip it halfway through. When done, shift to a serving plate and serve.

Per serving:

Calories 755 | Total Fat 57.6g 74% | Total Carbohydrate 19.1g 7% | Dietary Fiber 2g 7% | Protein 36.5g

— Steakhouse Steak —

Prep: 12 Minutes | Cook Time: 10-12 Minutes | Makes: 2 Servings

Spices Ingredients:

- 4 tablespoons of olive oil
- 2 clove Garlic
- 1 tablespoon tarragon
- ½ tablespoon rosemary
- Salt and black pepper, to taste
- ½ teaspoon Dijon mustard
- 2 teaspoons of lemon juice

Meat Ingredients:

- 1 pound (450gr) rib-eye steak, boneless

Directions:

1. Start by preheating the air fryer to around 400 ° F (205°C) before cooking for 4 minutes. Add all the listed spices to a bowl and mix them well. Add the steak to the bowl and rub the spice around it, letting it rest for at least 30 minutes.
2. Once the steak has rested in the marinade for enough time, shift it in the air fryer basket and cook it for around 10-12 minutes at 400 ° F (205°C), making sure to flip it halfway while cooking. When done, take it out and serve.

Per serving:

Calories 954 | Total Fat 82.3g 10 6% | Total Carbohydrate 2.2g 1% | Dietary Fiber 0.6g 2% | Protein 57.2g

— Pork Bites 2 —

Prep: 15 Minutes | Cook Time: 6 Minutes | Makes: 3 Servings

Ingredients:

- 1.5 pounds (680gr) of pork tenderloin
- 2 tablespoons olive oil
- 2 tablespoons Cajun seasoning

Directions:

1. Start by preheating the air fryer to around 400 ° F (205°C). Dice the pork into bite-size cubes and place it in a bowl. Add oil to the bowl and toss the cubes in it. Then season them with Cajun seasoning and shift them to the air fryer basket, cooking them for around 6 minutes at 400 ° F (205°C). Once the internal temperature reaches around 145 ° F (60°C), take them out and serve.

Per serving:

Calories 404| Total Fat 17.3g 22%| Total Carbohydrate 0g 0%| Dietary Fiber 0g 0%| Protein 59.4g

— Jalapeno Pepper Bake Pork —

Prep: 20 Minutes | Cook Time: 12 Minutes | Makes: 2 Servings

Ingredients:

- ¼ cup lime juice
- 2 tablespoons olive oil
- ½ teaspoon ground cumin
- 2 garlic cloves, minced
- ½ teaspoon dried oregano
- 1.5 pounds (680gr) pork tenderloin, ¾ inch slices

Pepper Mix Ingredients:

- 2 jalapeno peppers, seeded and chopped
- 2 tablespoons lime juice
- 2 teaspoons of stevia, Salt and black pepper
- ½ cup chopped red onion
- ½ tablespoon chopped mint
- 2 tablespoons lime zest, grated
- Salt and black pepper, to taste

Directions:

1. Add lime juice, olive oil, cumin, garlic, and oregano in a bowl. Once mixed, coat the pork tenderloin with it and let it rest in the marinade for at least 20 minutes. In another bowl, add all the listed ingredients for the pepper mix.
2. Once the pork has rested, shift it into the air fryer basket greased with oil spray, and cook it at 400 ° F (205°C) for 12-14 minutes (135 ° F (55°C) on a thermometer).When done, shift the pork to a serving dish and serve it with a side of pepper mix.

Per serving:

Calories 315 | Total Fat 13.1g 17% | Total Carbohydrate 2.6g 1% | Dietary Fiber 0.8g 3% | Protein 44.9g

— Steak and Vegetable —

Prep: 12 Minutes | Cook Time: 16 Minutes | Makes: 4 Servings

Sauce Ingredients:

- 2 cloves garlic, minced
- 1 tablespoon grated ginger-garlic paste
- ¼ teaspoon red chili flakes
- ¼ cup coconut amino
- ¼ cup rice vinegar, ½ cup stevia
- 2 teaspoons sesame oil
- 2 teaspoons of five spices

Steak Ingredients:

- 2 pounds (900gr) of sirloin steak

Directions:

1. Add all the listed sauce ingredients to a bowl and mix them. Once mixed, add the steak to the mixture and toss it around to coat the edges evenly. Once marinated, sift the steak to the basket of an air fryer lined with parchment paper, and cook it for around 8-12 minutes (medium rare) at about 400 ° F (205°C). When done, take it out and let it rest before serving.

Per serving:

Calories 479 | Total Fat 18.6g 24% | Total Carbohydrate 1.6g 1% | Dietary Fiber 0g 0% | Protein 69.1g

— Pork Meat and Cabbage Rolls —

Prep: 20 Minutes | Cook Time: 6-8 Minutes| Makes: 2 Servings

Ingredients:

- ½ cup stewed cabbage
- 5 tablespoons of spicy mustard
- 1 cup of pork meat, shredded, cooked, and boneless
- 6 coconut wraps, Oil spray for greasing

Directions:

1. Start by mixing cabbage, mustard, and meat in a bowl. Place the wraps onto a clean and flat surface. Equally, distribute the mixture to the wraps and roll.
2. Mist the rolls with oil spray and place them in the air fryer basket lined with parchment paper, cooking them for around 6-8 minutes at about 400 ° F (205°C). Make sure to flip them halfway while cooking. Once done, serve.

Per serving:

Calories 692 | Total Fat 31.8g 41% | Total Carbohydrate 24g 9% | Dietary Fiber 3g 11% | Protein 66g

⚊ Sticky Beef Ribs ⚊

Prep: 10 Minutes | Cook Time: 20 Minutes | Makes: 4 Servings

Ingredients:

- 4 beef short ribs, flanked cut
- 1 teaspoon garlic, minced
- 2 tablespoons olive oil
- 2 tablespoons Vegan mushroom sauce
- 2 teaspoon sesame oil

Directions:

1. Start by preheating the air fryer before cooking to around 400 ° F (205°C). Place the beef ribs in a bowl and add all the listed ingredients over it, mixing and messaging them on the ribs.
2. Once coated, shift it to the air fryer basket and cook it for around 20 minutes at about 400 ° F (205°C). When done, move the ribs to a serving plate and serve.

Per serving:

Calories 1294| Total Fat 68.3g 88%| Total Carbohydrate 0.5g 0%| Dietary Fiber 0g 0%|Protein 159.5g

⚊ Pepper Sirloin Steak ⚊

Prep: 10 Minutes | Cook Time: 8 Minutes | Makes: 2 Servings

Ingredients:

- 2 tablespoons of olive oil
- 2 sirloin steaks, 8 ounces (230gr) each
- Salt and black pepper, to taste
- Oil spray for greasing

Blue cheese butter Ingredients:

- 4 teaspoons unsalted butter
- 3-4 ounces (100gr) of blue cheese
- ¼ cup parsley, chopped
- ¼ cup of thyme, chopped
- ¼ cup of rosemary, chopped
- ¼ cup of chives, chopped
- 4 minced garlic cloves

Directions:

1. Drizzle oil over the steak and season it with salt and pepper. Grease the basket of air fryer with oil and place the steak in it, cooking it for 8 minutes at 390 °F (200°C), flipping halfway through (it gives medium rare). Note: Take out at 125 ° F (50°C) internal temperature for the medium-rare result. Flip the steak halfway to ensure an even cook throughout.
2. Meanwhile, combine all the blue cheese ingredients and top it over the steak once taken out from the basket. Enjoy.

Per serving:

Calories 815 | Total Fat 49.9g 64% | Total Carbohydrate 12.2g 4% | Dietary Fiber 5.8g 21% | Protein 79.7g

⚊ Cheese-Filled Beef Roll-Ups ⚊

Prep: 22 Minutes | Cook Time: 16 Minutes | Makes: 2 Servings

Ingredients:

- 1.2 pounds (550gr) of flank steaks, butterflied
- ½ cup Swiss cheese
- ½ cup ounces of sauerkraut
- 2 tablespoons of bagel seasoning, as needed
- Oil spray for greasing
- Salt and black pepper, to taste

Directions:

1. Start by preheating the air fryer to around 400 ° F (205°C). Place the butterflied steak onto a clean surface, top it with the cheese, sauerkraut, and seasoning, rectangle and roll over the edges, and secure with kitchen twine. Drizzle the oil over it and season it with salt and pepper.
2. Put it into the air fryer basket, cooking them for around 16 minutes at about 400 ° F (205°C), flipping halfway. When done, take them out and serve.

Per serving:

Calories 633| Total Fat 30.4g 39%| Total Carbohydrate 1.5g 1%| Dietary Fiber 0g 0%|Protein 83g

⚊ Garlic Herb Butter Rib Eye ⚊

Prep: 12 Minutes | Cook Time: 12 Minutes | Makes: 4 Servings

Garlic Herb Butter Ingredients:

- ½ cup softened butter
- 4 garlic cloves, minced
- ½ teaspoon fresh rosemary
- ½ teaspoon fresh thyme
- ½ teaspoon fresh parsley

Steak Ingredients:

- 2 rib-eye, 1 inch (25mm) thick each
- 2 teaspoons Italian seasoning
- 4 tablespoons olive oil, Salt and pepper, to taste

Directions:

1. Start by preheating the air fryer to around 400 ° F (205°C) before cooking. Add all the garlic herb butter ingredients in a bowl and mix. Season all the sides of the steak with salt, pepper, and Italian seasoning. Coat the steaks with olive oil as well.
2. Once seasoned, shift it to the air fryer basket and cook it for around 12 minutes at 400 ° F (205°C), making sure to flip it halfway. When done, shift it to a serving plate and serve it with the herb butter made earlier.

Per serving:

Calories 569 | Total Fat 56.6g 73% | Total Carbohydrate 1.5g 1% | Dietary Fiber 0.2g 1% | Protein 15.5g

Mustard and Rosemary Rib Eye Steak

Prep: 16 Minutes | Cook Time: 16 Minutes | Makes: 4 Servings

Ingredients:
- 2 tablespoons of apple cider vinegar
- ½ cup Dijon mustard, Salt and black pepper, to taste
- 2 teaspoons rosemary
- 2 tablespoons of olive oil
- 1.5 pounds (680gr) Rib eye steak, cubed

Directions:
1. Add apple cider vinegar, mustard, rosemary, salt, and pepper in a bowl. Drizzle oil over the steak and season it with a bowl of ingredients.
2. Shift it to the air fryer and cook it for around 16 minutes at 400°F (205°C), flipping halfway through. When done, take it out and let it rest before serving.

Per serving:

Calories 551 | Total Fat 46g 59% | Total Carbohydrate 2.1g 1% | Dietary Fiber 1.3g 5% | Protein 31.5g

Rib Eye with Zucchini Noodles

Prep: 22 Minutes | Cook Time: 25 Minutes | Makes: 4 Servings

Ingredients:
- 1.5 cups zucchini noodles, cooked
- ½ tablespoon paprika
- 1 teaspoon caraway seeds
- Salt and black pepper, to taste
- 4 tablespoons of olive oil
- 12 ounces (340gr) rib eye steak, cubed
- 1 teaspoon of thyme
- 1 teaspoon of rosemary
- 1 cup sour cream

Directions:
1. Start by cutting 3 zucchini into spirals resembling noodles and place them in water, boiling them till tender and soft. Once done, drain them. Add paprika, caraway seeds, salt, and pepper to a bowl.
2. Drizzle oil over the steak, season it with thyme and rosemary and bowl the seasoning mix.
3. Shift it to an air fryer basket lined with parchment paper, cooking it at around 400 ° F (205°C) for about 16 minutes, flipping it after 8 minutes. When it's done, take it out and let it rest. Once rested, cube it and serve it over sour cream and zucchini noodles.

Per serving:

Calories 488 | Total Fat 45.1g 5 8% | Total Carbohydrate 4.9g 2% | Dietary Fiber 1.2g 4% | Protein 17.4g

Rump Steak

Prep: 10 Minutes | Cook Time: 16-18 Minutes | Makes: 3 Servings

Ingredients:
- 2 tablespoons of avocado oil
- 1.5 pounds (680gr) of rump steak
- 4 tablespoons of steak seasoning
- Oil spray for greasing

Directions:
1. Start by drizzling oil over the steak and rubbing it around.
2. Then season it with steak seasoning and shift it to the air fryer basket greased with oil spray, cooking it for about 400°F (205°C) for 16-18 minutes, making sure to flip after 8 minutes of cooking.
3. When done, serve and enjoy.

Per serving:

Calories 420| Total Fat 15g 19%| Total Carbohydrate 0.5g 0%| Dietary Fiber 0.4g 1%| Protein 70.4g

Bourbon Lamb Chops

Prep: 20 Minutes | Cook Time: 14 Minutes | Makes: 2Servings

Ingredients for marinade:
- 1 tablespoon dry mustard powder
- 1 tablespoon stevia
- ½ cup bourbon
- 1 tablespoon Worcestershire sauce, sugar-free
- 1 tablespoon soy sauce
- 2 tablespoons balsamic vinegar
- Salt and black pepper to taste

Other Ingredients:
- 6 boneless pork chops

Directions:
1. Start by mixing all the ingredients listed for the marinade in a bowl, adding the chops, and coating them completely. Let the coated chops rest in the fridge for at least 1 hour.
2. Once they have rested for enough time, shift them to an air fryer basket lined with foil and cook them for at least 12-16 minutes at around 400 ° F (205°C). Baste the chops with sauce halfway. Make sure to flip them after 7 minutes.
3. Meanwhile, reduce the remaining sauce in the saucepan by simmering it for a few minutes. When done, serve chops with an additional sauce.

Per serving:

Calories 830| Total Fat 40.6g 52%| Total Carbohydrate 7.2g 3%| Dietary Fiber 0.9g 3%| Protein 76.9g

Garlic Rosemary Pork Chops with Blue Cheese Butter

Prep: 15 Minutes | Cook Time: 12 Minutes | Makes: 4 Servings

Ingredients:

- 4 tablespoons of olive oil
- Salt and black pepper, to taste
- 2 rosemary leaves
- ½ teaspoon of fresh thyme, chopped
- 4 tablespoons of butter
- 2 cloves of garlic cloves
- 6 pork chops

Side serving:

- 1 cup blue cheese, ½ cup butter

Directions:

1. Add oil, salt, pepper, rosemary, thyme, butter, and garlic clove in a high-speed blender until they turn into a paste. Place the chops in a bowl and add the paste on top, coating it around the chops and letting it rest in the fridge for at least 1 hour.
2. Once it has rested for enough time, grease the basket with oil spray, and place the pork chop in it, cooking it for around 8-12 minutes at about 360 ° F (180°C).
3. Mix blue cheese with butter and top it over cooked chops. Serve it hot.

Per serving:

Calories 917 | Total Fat 81.3g 10 4% | Total Carbohydrate 7.8g 3% | Dietary Fiber 2g 7% | Protein 42.5g

Easy Steak Bites

Prep: 12 Minutes | Cook Time: 6 Minutes | Makes: 2 Servings

Ingredients:

- 1 lb (450gr) of sirloin steak, cut into bite-size pieces
- 2 teaspoons of olive oil, as needed
- 1 tablespoon Steak seasoning
- Salt and pepper, to taste

Directions:

1. Start by preheating the air fryer before cooking to around 400 ° F (205°C) for 5 minutes. Add the steak bites to a bowl, drizzle olive oil over them, and season them with steak seasoning, salt, and pepper.
2. Once coated, add the steak bits to the basket of the air fryer in a single layer and cook them for around 6 minutes at 400°F (205°C), tossing the basket halfway.
3. When done, take them out of the air fryer and let them rest for at least 4 minutes before serving them.

Per serving:

Calories 461 | Total Fat 18.8g 24% | Total Carbohydrate 0g 0% | Dietary Fiber 0g 0% | Protein 68.8g

Spicy Beef Tenderloin

Prep: 15 minutes | cook time: 15-20 minutes | makes: 3 servings

Ingredients:

- 4 teaspoons of lemon juice
- 2 pounds (900gr) of beef tenderloin
- Salt and black pepper, to taste
- 1 teaspoon of rosemary, dried
- 1 teaspoon of thyme, dried
- 4 tablespoons of butter, melted
- Oil spray for greasing

Directions:

1. Start by drizzling lemon juice over the beef tenderloin and seasoning it with salt, pepper, rosemary, and thyme. Rub butter all over.
2. Once seasoned, shift it to the basket of air fryer lined with parchment paper, cook it for around 15-20 minutes at 380°F (195°C), and flip the tenderloin halfway.
3. When done, take the steak out. Let it rest for 4 minutes before serving.

Per serving:

Calories 764 | Total Fat 43.3g 56% |Total Carbohydrate 0.6g 0% | Dietary Fiber 0.3g 1% | Protein 87.8g

Tri Tip Garlic Butter Glazed Steak

Prep: 12 Minutes | Cook Time: 16 Minutes | Makes: 2 Servings

Ingredients:

- Salt and black pepper, to taste
- ¼ cup soy sauce
- 2 teaspoons of olive oil
- 1/3 teaspoon of grated ginger
- 4 cloves garlic, minced
- 1-½ tablespoons of stevia
- 2 tri-tip steaks
- Oil spray for greasing
- 6 tablespoons of garlic butter, solid

Directions:

1. Start by adding salt, pepper, soy sauce, olive oil, ginger, garlic, and stevia in a bowl and mixing them. Then place the steak in it and coat it well. Shift it to the fridge and let it rest for at least 1 hour.
2. Once marinated, shift it in the air fryer basket greased with oil spray, and cook it at around 400 ° F (205°C) for 12 minutes, flipping halfway. When done, remove the steak and top it with garlic butter.

Per serving:

Calories 1417 | Total Fat 87.1g 112% | Total Carbohydrate 4.7g 2% | Dietary Fiber 0.4g 2% | Protein 154.6g

Pork Chops with Horseradish Sauce

Prep: 12 Minutes | Cook Time: 8-12 Minutes | Makes: 2 Servings

Horseradish Sauce Ingredients:

- ½ cup mayonnaise
- 2 tablespoons Dijon mustard
- 1 tablespoon prepared horseradish
- 2 tablespoons stevia

Pork Chop Ingredients:

- 6 pork chops
- 4 tablespoons vegetable oil
- 4 cloves garlic, minced
- Salt and black pepper, to taste
- Oil spray for greasing

Directions:

1. Mix all the required ingredients for the Horseradish sauce in a bowl. Season the pork chops with vegetable oil, garlic, salt, and black pepper.
2. Grease the basket of air fryer with oil spray, place the pork chops according to capacity and cook it for around 8-12 minutes at about 360 ° F (180°C). Make sure to flip halfway in the cooking to ensure an even cook throughout.
3. When done, shift them to a serving plate and serve them with the sauce made earlier.

Per serving:

Calories 842 | Total Fat 71.6g 92% | Total Carbohydrate 11.8g 4% | Dietary Fiber 0.6g 2% | Protein 37.1g

Easy Boston Butt

Prep: 10 Minutes | Cook Time: 50 Minutes | Makes: 4 Servings

Ingredients:

- 1 teaspoon of ground clove
- 1 teaspoon of ground ginger
- 4 tablespoons of avocado oil
- 1/6 teaspoon of cinnamon
- Salt and black pepper, to taste
- 2 pounds (900gr) Boston butt

Directions:

1. Add all the ingredients listed in a bowl and mix them. Rub the Boston butt with the prepared mixture. Place it indie the fridge and let it rest for at least 10 minutes.
2. Once it has rested for enough time, shift it to the air fryer basket greased with oil spray, and cook it for around 50 minutes at about 360 ° F (180°C). When done, shift it to a serving bowl and serve.

Per serving:

Calories 610 | Total Fat 39.6g 51% | Total Carbohydrate 1.5g 1% | Dietary Fiber 0.9g 3% | Protein 58.3g

Chipotle New York Steak

Prep: 10 Minutes | Cook Time: 12 Minutes | Makes: 1 Serving

Ingredients:

- 2 New York steaks, 1 pound (450gr)
- 2 tablespoons of olive oil
- 1 tablespoon chipotle seasoning, no sugar
- 1 tablespoon stevia
- 1/3 teaspoon cumin
- Oil spray for greasing

Directions:

1. Start by preheating the air fryer to around 400 ° F (205°C) before cooking for 5 minutes. Drizzle oil over the steak, rub it around, then season it with chipotle powder, stevia, and cumin, and set it aside once fully coated for a few minutes.
2. Grease the basket of air fryer with oil spray, and add the steak to it, cooking it for around 6-8 minutes on each side at 400 ° F (205°C). When done, shift the steak to a serving plate and serve.

Per serving:

Calories 781 | Total Fat 28.7g 37% | Total Carbohydrate 133.7g 49% | Dietary Fiber 0.1g 0% | Protein 0.1g

Classic Style Ribs

Prep: 12 Minutes | Cook Time: 28-32 Minutes | Makes: 6 Servings

Rub Ingredients:

- 4 tablespoons olive oil
- 2 teaspoons dry mustard
- 1 teaspoon thyme
- 1 teaspoon garlic powder
- ½ teaspoon dried marjoram
- Salt and black pepper, to taste

Pork ribs Ingredients:

- 3 -4 pounds (1700gr) of baby back pork ribs, cut into 4 equal portions

Directions:

1. Start by preheating the air fryer to around 380 ° F (195°C) for 5 minutes before starting the cooking. Add all the ingredients for the rub in a bowl and mix them, rubbing it over the ribs once mixed and letting the ribs rest in the fridge for at least 60 minutes.
2. When done, shift the pork ribs to the air fryer basket and cook them for around 28-32 minutes, making sure to flip them after 10 minutes each at 350°F (180°C).
3. When it's done, remove it from the basket and let it rest for some time before serving.

Per serving:

Calories 707 | Total Fat 49.8g 64% | Total Carbohydrate 0.9g 0% | Dietary Fiber 0.3g 1% | Protein 60.5g

Rosemary Garlic Lamb Chops

Prep: 20 Minutes | Cook Time: 8-12 Minutes | Makes: 3 Servings

Ingredients:

- 1.5 pounds (680gr) rack of lamb, about 7-8 chops
- 4 teaspoons olive oil
- 4 teaspoons chopped fresh rosemary
- 1 teaspoon garlic powder
- Salt and black pepper, to taste

Directions:

1. Start by patting dry the lamb racks and cleaning any excess fat. Cut the chops into smaller pieces. Mix olive oil, rosemary, garlic, salt, and pepper in a bowl and coat the lamb. Cover it and let it stay there for at least 1 hour or overnight if available.
2. Preheat the air fryer to around 390 ° F (200°C) for at least 4 minutes before cooking the chops. Once the air fryer is preheated, and the chops are marinated for enough time, shift to the basket and air fry for around 6 minutes at 400 ° F (205°C), flipping halfway. Cook for 2-4 minutes more at 400 ° F (205°C).

Per serving:

Calories 822 | Total Fat 50.2g 64% | Total Carbohydrate 2.6g 1% | Dietary Fiber 1.2g 4% | Protein 85.4g

— Perfect Pork Ribs —

Prep: 10 Minutes | Cook Time: 22-25 Minutes | Makes: 4 Servings

Ingredients:

- 3 pounds (1350gr) of baby pork ribs, quartered
- 2 tablespoons almond flour
- 2 tablespoons coconut oil
- ¼teaspoon dry mustard
- ¼teaspoon garlic powder
- ¼teaspoon dried marjoram
- Salt and black pepper, to taste
- Oil spray for greasing

Directions:

1. Start by preheating the air fryer to around 380 ° F (195°C) for at least 2 minutes before cooking. Mix all the listed ingredients in a bowl and shift the bowl to the fridge, letting it rest for at least 2 hours.
2. Once the pork ribs have rested for enough time, grease the inside of the air fryer basket with oil and place them in it, cooking them for around 22-25 minutes at 380 ° F (195°C). Make sure to flip them halfway. Take them out once done and serve.

Per serving:

Calories 1030 | Total Fat 88.7g 114% | Total Carbohydrate 0.4g 0% | Dietary Fiber 0.2g 1% | Protein 54.5g

— Blueberry Pork Tenderloin —

Prep: 12 Minutes | Cook Time: 22 Minutes | Makes: 2 Servings

Ingredients:

- 2 tablespoons of olive oil
- 1 .5 pounds (680gr) of pork tenderloin
- Salt and black pepper, to taste
- ¼ cup of stevia
- ½ cup blueberries
- 1 large onion, peeled
- Oil spray

Directions:

1. Start by drizzling oil over the tenderloin, massaging it, and seasoning the pork with salt, pepper, and stevia.
2. Mix berries and onions in a bowl and season them accordingly with salt and pepper and mist with oil spray.
3. Shift the blueberries and onions into the basket lined with parchment paper, top them with the pork tenderloin, and cook them together for around 22 minutes at about 400°F (205°C).
4. When done, shift them to a serving plate and serve. Note: Internal temperature at the end should be 145° – 165°F (60-75°C).

Per serving:

Calories 336 | Total Fat 18.5g 24% | Total Carbohydrate 12.3g 4% | Dietary Fiber 2.5g 9% | Protein 30.8g

— Mojito Spiced Chop —

Prep: 20 Minutes | Cook Time: 12 Minutes | Makes: 2 Servings

Ingredients:

- 2 lemons, juice only
- Salt, to taste
- ½ cup mint leaves
- 1/3 cup olive oil
- 4 large cloves garlic, minced
- 6 lamb chops, trimmed

Directions:

1. Start by mixing lemon juice, salt, mint leaves, oil, and Garlic in a blender until a smooth paste is formed. Pour this paste over the lamb and coat it, letting it stays in the fridge for at least 30 minutes.
2. Then shift it to the air fryer basket lined with foil, and cook it for around 12 minutes at about 400 ° F (205°C). Make sure to flip the ribs halfway while cooking and serve when done.

Per serving:

Calories 1072| Total Fat 97.7g 125%| Total Carbohydrate 1.9g 1%| Dietary Fiber 1.6g 6%| Protein 50.9g

— Minty Yogurt Chops —

Prep: 15 Minutes | Cook Time: 16 Minutes | Makes: 4 Servings

Ingredients:

- 2 tablespoons of lemon juice
- 1 cup plain yogurt
- ¼ cup parsley, chopped
- ½ cup mint, chopped
- 1 teaspoon of five-spice powder
- Salt and black pepper, to taste
- ½ teaspoon of ginger garlic paste
- 8 lamb chops
- Oil spray for greasing

Directions:

1. Start by adding all the ingredients except the lambs and blending them in a blender. Pour the sauce over the lambs and let them rest in the fridge, marinated for at least a few hours.
2. Once rested, shift the lamb to the air fryer basket lined with aluminum foil and cook it for around 16 minutes at about 350 ° F (180°C), flipping halfway. Once it's done, serve.

Per serving:

Calories 569| Total Fat 43.7g 56%| Total Carbohydrate 5.7g 2%| Dietary Fiber 0.9g 3%| Protein 37.4g

— Pork Chops —

Prep: 20 Minutes | Cook Time: 12-14 Minutes | Makes: 3 Servings

Ingredients:

- 2 tablespoons almond flour
- 1 teaspoon smoked paprika
- 1 tablespoon of olive oil
- 2 tablespoons white wine vinegar
- 2 teaspoons soy sauce
- Salt and black pepper, to taste
- 2 teaspoons Dijon mustard
- 6 bone-in thick-cut pork chops

Directions:

1. Start by preheating the air fryer to around 400 ° F (205°C) before cooking. Add all the listed ingredients in a bowl and mix them. Add the chops to the bowl and coat them with the marinade.
2. Once coated, shift them to the air fryer basket and cook them for around 16 minutes at 400 ° F (205°C). Flip the chops halfway through to ensure an even cook throughout. When done, serve and enjoy.

Per serving:

Calories 309 | Total Fat 18.8g 24% | Total Carbohydrate 1.7g 1% | Dietary Fiber 0.3g 1% | Protein 34.4g

— Pesto Steak —

Prep: 22 Minutes | Cook Time: 6 Minutes | Makes: 2 Servings

Ingredients:

- 2 tablespoons of olive oil
- 2 lamb steaks, 1 pound (450gr) approx
- Salt and black pepper, to taste

Salad ingredients:

- 1 cup feta cheese, crumbled
- 6 ounces (170gr) baby spinach, chopped
- ½ cup walnuts, chopped
- 1 cup grape tomatoes, halved

Directions:

1. Start by preheating the air fryer to around 400 ° F (205°C) for at least 2 minutes before cooking. Drizzle oil over the lamb steaks and season them with salt and pepper.
2. Once seasoned, shift them to the air fryer basket and cook them for around 6 minutes (medium rare) at 400 ° F (205°C), making sure to flip them halfway while cooking.
3. Mix cheese, spinach, walnuts, and tomatoes in a bowl and drizzle with olive oil. Add the steak on it once over the top of the salad and serve.

Per serving:

Calories 855| Total Fat 60.3g 77%| Total Carbohydrate 12.8g 5%| Dietary Fiber 5.1g 18%| Protein 69g

— Beef Back Ribs —

Prep: 20 Minutes | Cook Time: 25 Minutes | Makes: 4 Servings

Ingredients:

- 1 cup of BBQ sauce, keto-based and unsweetened
- 2 pounds (900gr) of beef back ribs, cut in thirds
- Salt and black pepper, to taste
- Oil spray for greasing

Directions:

1. Start by preheating the air fryer to around 400 ° F (205°C) for at least 2 minutes before cooking. Add half of the BBQ sauce over the beef ribs and coat them. Then season the ribs with salt and pepper.
2. Place the ribs in the basket of air fryer greased with oil spray, and cook them for around 18-20 minutes at about 375 ° F (190°C), flipping halfway through.
3. Baste the ribs with the remaining BBQ sauce and cook for 5 more minutes. When done, shift them to a serving plate and serve.

Per serving:

Calories 601 | Total Fat 28g 36% | Total Carbohydrate 22.7g 8% | Dietary Fiber 0.4g 1% | Protein 59.7g

Marinated Lamb Chops

Prep: 20 Minutes | Cook Time: 8-12 Minutes | Makes: 3 Servings

Ingredients:

- 1.5 pounds (680gr) of lamb chops

Marinade Ingredients:

- 2 tablespoons olive oil
- 2 tablespoons red wine vinegar
- 1 teaspoon dried rosemary
- ½ teaspoon dried oregano
- Salt and black pepper, to taste
- ½ teaspoon garlic powder

Directions:

1. Start by mixing olive oil, red wine vinegar, rosemary, oregano, salt, pepper, and garlic powder in a bowl and place the lamb chops in it, and coat the chops, letting them stay coated for at least 1 hour.
2. Preheat the air fryer to around 400 ° F (205°C) for 6 minutes. Once preheated, shift the lamb chops to the air fryer basket and cook them for about 8-12 minutes at 400 ° F (205°C).

Per serving:

Calories 508 | Total Fat 26g 33% | Total Carbohydrate 0.9g 0% | Dietary Fiber 0.3g 1% | Protein 63.8g

Juicy vegetables and Sirloin Steak with Sour Cream

Prep: 12 Minutes | Cook Time: 12 Minutes | Makes: 3 Servings

Ingredients:

- 1.5 pounds (680gr) beef sirloin steak,cut into strips
- ¼ cup beef broth
- 6 ounces green beans, halved
- ½ cup diced tomatoes, undrained
- 6 ounces (170gr) of frozen pearl onions, thawed
- 1 tablespoon paprika
- Salt and black pepper, to taste
- 1 cup sour cream
- Oil spray for greasing

Directions:

1. Start by preheating the air fryer to around 400 ° F (205°C) for 5 minutes. Add the steak bits, broths, green beans, tomatoes, onions, paprika, salt, and pepper in a bowl. Grease the air fryer basket with oil spray and shift everything in the basket, cooking them for around 12 minutes at 400 ° F (205°C).
2. When done, let the steak rest in the broth for around 5 to 10 minutes before serving it with sour cream.

Per serving:

Calories 640 | Total Fat 30.9g 40% | Total Carbohydrate 13.5g 5% | Dietary Fiber 4.2g 15% | Protein 74.6g

Hearty Lamb Chops Tomatina

Prep: 22 Minutes | Cook Time: 12 Minutes | Makes: 4 Servings

Ingredients:

- 6 plum tomatoes
- 3/4 cup vinegar
- 4 tablespoons olive oil
- Salt and pepper, to taste
- 4 garlic cloves, minced
- ¼ cup fresh basil leaves
- 8 lamb loin chops, boneless and cubed

Directions:

1. Add tomatoes, vinegar, olive oil, salt, pepper, garlic cloves, and basils in a blender until they form a smooth paste. Coat the lambs with the paste and let it rest and refrigerator for at least 1 hour.
2. Once rested, shift it to an air fryer basket lined with foil, and cook it for 12-16 minutes at around 400 ° F (205°C), making sure to flip it halfway while cooking. When done, take them out and serve.

Per serving:

Calories 957| Total Fat 52.1g 67%| Total Carbohydrate 10.9g 4%| Dietary Fiber 2.1g 8%| Protein 105.1g

Boneless Pork Chops

Prep: 15 Minutes | Cook Time: 12-14 Minutes | Makes: 4 Servings

Meat Ingredients:

- 2 pounds (900gr) of boneless pork chops
- Oil spray for greasing

Marinade Ingredients:

- 4 tablespoons of soy sauce
- ¼ cup red wine
- 4 tablespoons of fish sauce
- 4 tablespoons of hoisin sauce
- 2 teaspoons stevia
- 2 teaspoons of ginger garlic, paste
- 2 teaspoons of five-spice powder
- Salt and black pepper, to taste

Directions:

1. Mix all the ingredients for the marinade in a bowl, add the pork chops, and let it rest for 1 hour in the refrigerator. Once the pork has rested, grease the inside of the air fryer basket with oil spray and place the pork chop there, cooking it for around 12-14 minutes at 400 ° F (205°C) making sure to flip them halfway while cooking. When done, shift them to a serving plate and serve.

Per serving:

Calories 387| Total Fat 8.5g 11%| Total Carbohydrate 9.4g 3%| Dietary Fiber 0.6g 2%| Protein 61.8g

— Classic Pork Chops —

Prep: 18 Minutes | Cook Time: 12-14 Minutes | Makes: 2 Servings

Ingredients:

- 4 tablespoons olive oil
- Salt, to taste
- 1 teaspoon smoked paprika
- 1 tablespoon dry oregano
- 1 tablespoon of dry thyme
- 1 teaspoon of cayenne pepper
- 1 tablespoon garlic powder
- 2 pounds (900gr) of boneless pork chops

Directions:

1. Add olive oil and listed seasoning in a bowl and mix them. Once mixed, coat the pork chops with the seasoning, covering all the corners once mixed.

2. Preheat the air fryer for 6 minutes before cooking at 400 ° F (205°C). Put the pork chop in the air fryer basket greased with oil spray, and cook it for around 12-14 minutes at 400 ° F (205°C). Make sure to flip the chops halfway through the cooking.

3. Once the internal temperature reaches around 135 ° F (55°C), take it out and shift it to a serving plate and serve. Let it rest for 10 minutes and serve.

Per serving:

Calories 919 | Total Fat 44.6g 57% |Total Carbohydrate 6.5g 2% | Dietary Fiber 2.5g 9% | Protein 120g

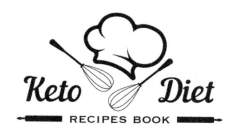

Chapter

9

Fish and Seafood

⸺ Fish Fillet with Onion Rings ⸺

Prep: 10 Minutes | Cook Time: 14 Minutes | Makes: 4 Servings

Ingredients:
- 2 codfish fillets, 6 ounces (170gr) each
- 2 teaspoons of lemon juice
- Salt and black pepper, to taste
- 1 cup of onion, cut into rings
- ½ cup almond flour
- 1 teaspoon paprika
- salt and black pepper, to taste
- 1/3 cup pork rinds, grated
- oil spray for greasing

Directions:
1. Start by patting dry the fillet using a paper towel. Then drizzle lemon juice onto fillets and season it with salt and pepper. Coat the onions with almond flour, paprika, salt, pepper, and pork rinds.
2. Grease the inside of the air fryer with oil and place the fish in it. Arrange the onion rings beside the codfish fillet, and cook it for around 14 minutes at about 350°F (180°C). When done, shift them to a serving bowl and serve.

Per serving:

Calories 534 | Total Fat 24.9g 32% | Total Carbohydrate 3.8g 1% | Dietary Fiber 1.2g 4%| Protein 70.3g

⸺ Divine Salmon ⸺

Prep: 25 Minutes | Cook Time: 14 Minutes | Makes: 2 Servings

Ingredients:
- 1/3 cup tamari sauce
- ¼ cup water
- 4 cloves of garlic, minced
- 4 tablespoons sesame oil
- 4 teaspoons sesame seeds
- ½ tablespoon ginger, grated
- ½ tablespoon stevia
- 1/3 cup whole wine vinegar
- 20 ounces (570gr) of salmon fillets, 2 pieces

Directions:
1. Mix tamari sauce, water, garlic, sesame oil, seeds, ginger, stevia, and white wine vinegar in a bowl. Once everything is dissolved, add the fish to the bowl and coat it with everything. Let the fish stay in the marinade for at least 30 minutes.
2. Cover the fish with foil and place it in the air fryer basket cooking it for around 12 minutes at about 370°F (190°C). Flip the fish halfway in the cooking to ensure even cooking.
3. Once cooked for 12 minutes, remove the foil and cook it for another 2 minutes. When done, shift the fish to a serving plate and serve.

Per serving:

Calories 663 | Total Fat 47.8g 61% | Total Carbohydrate 4.4g 2% | Dietary Fiber 1g 4% | Protein 56.6g

— Crab and Mushrooms —

Prep: 12 Minutes | Cook Time: 9-10 Minutes | Makes: 2 Servings

Ingredients:

- 4 ounces (115gr) mushrooms

For Stuffing:

- 4 ounces (115gr) chopped crab meat
- 1 green onion, finely chopped
- 1/8 cup mayo
- ¼ cup Parmesan cheese
- 1 teaspoon parsley
- ¼ teaspoon paprika
- salt and black Pepper to taste

Directions:

1. Start by preheating the air fryer to around 380 ° F (195°C). Wash the mushrooms with water and remove the stems and gills. Line the bottom of the basket of the air fryer with foil. Add the ingredients for the stuffing in a bowl and mix them. Take a spoonful of the mixture and fill the mushrooms with it. Mist the mushroom with oil spray.
2. Arrange the mushrooms in the air fryer basket lined with foil in a single layer and cook them for at least 9 minutes at 400 ° F (205°C). Once done, serve.

Per serving:

Calories 214 | Total Fat 12.1g 16% | Total Carbohydrate 8.1g 3% | Dietary Fiber 0.9g 3% | Protein 18.2g

— Salmon with Coconut —

Prep: 15 Minutes | Cook Time: 12 Minutes | Makes: 2 Servings

Ingredients:

- Salt and ground black pepper, to taste
- 3 tablespoons organic butter
- 1 tablespoon red curry paste
- 1 cup of coconut cream
- 2 salmon fillets, 6 ounces (170gr) each
- ½ cup Parmesan cheese

Directions:

1. Preheat the unit to 390 ° F (200°C) before cooking, for a few minutes before cooking. Start by mixing salt, pepper, butter, red curry paste, and coconut cream in a bowl and marinating the fish.
2. Line the bottom of the basket with parchment paper and place the salmon fillet on them, cooking them for around 12 minutes at 375 ° F (190°C). Flip the fish halfway in the cooking to ensure even cooking. When done, serve the fish with a garnish of cheese.

Per serving:

Calories 874 | Total Fat 71.1g 91% | Total Carbohydrate 10.2g 4% | Dietary Fiber 2.6g 9% | Protein 55.5g

— Spicy Shrimp —

Prep: 10 Minutes | Cook Time: 7 Minutes | Makes: 2 Servings

Ingredients:

- 1 teaspoon chili powder
- ½ teaspoon paprika powder
- ¼ teaspoon garlic powder
- ¼ teaspoon ground cayenne pepper
- ¼ teaspoon thyme
- ¼ teaspoon oregano
- Salt and black pepper to taste
- ¼ teaspoon cumin, 1 teaspoon olive oil
- ¼ teaspoon mustard
- 1 pound (450gr) shrimp

Directions:

1. Start by preheating the air fryer to around 400 ° F (205°C) for at least 5 minutes before cooking. Let the shrimp defrost, patting them dry using a paper towel once defrosted. Mix all the listed ingredients in a bowl and mix them. Coat the shrimp with olive oil or avocado oil and toss it in the spice mix.
2. Once seasoned, arrange them in the air fryer basket in a single layer and cook them for around 7 minutes at 400 ° F (205°C). When done, take them out and serve.

Per serving:

Calories 299 | Total Fat 6.6g 9% | Total Carbohydrate 5g 2% | Dietary Fiber 0.8g 3% | Protein 52.1g

— Cajun Salmon with Blue Cheese Dressing —

Prep: 15 Minutes | Cook Time: 8 Minutes | Makes: 2 Servings

Ingredients:

- 1 tablespoon of Cajun seasoning
- 1 tablespoon of jerk seasoning
- 4 tablespoons of lemon juice
- 2 tablespoons of olive oil
- 2 salmon fillets
- ½ cup blue cheese dressing

Directions:

1. Start by mixing Cajun spice, jerk seasoning, and lemon juice. Drizzle oil on both sides of the salmon fillet and season it with the seasoning mix.
2. Once seasoned, place it on the air fryer basket lined with aluminum foil and cook it for around 12 minutes at about 390 ° F (200°C), flipping the fish halfway through. When done, serve the fillet with a blue cheese dressing.

Per serving:

Calories 671 | Total Fat 57.3g 73% | Total Carbohydrate 5.2g 2% | Dietary Fiber 0.1g 0% | Protein 37.8g

― Breaded Sea Scallops ―

Prep: 15 Minutes | Cook Time: 6-8 Minutes | Makes: 2 Servings

Ingredients:

- 12 ounces (340gr) of sea scallops
- 4 teaspoons olive oil
- ½ teaspoon onion powder
- 1 teaspoon of Old Bay seasoning
- ½ teaspoon garlic powder
- Salt and black pepper, to taste
- ½ cup pork rinds, grated or pork Panko

Directions:

1. Place scallops in a bowl and drizzle olive oil on top. Add onion powder, oil, bay seasoning, garlic powder, salt, and pepper in another bowl. In another bowl, add pork rinds. Coat the scallops first with seasoning, then give them a coat of pork rinds
2. Once coated, shift them to the air fryer basket and cook them for around 6-8 minutes at about 400 ° F (205°C). Make sure to flip them halfway through the cooking. When done, take them out and serve.

Per serving:

Calories 347 | Total Fat 17.3g 22%vTotal Carbohydrate 5.4g 2% | Dietary Fiber 0.1g 0% | Protein 40.9g

― Salmon with Creamy Dill Sauce ―

Prep: 15 Minutes | Cook Time: 10 Minutes | Makes: 4 Servings

Ingredients for dill sauce:

- 1 cup low-fat plain Greek yogurt
- 1 teaspoon Dijon mustard
- 1 teaspoon lemon juice
- 2 tablespoons chopped dill

Salmon Ingredients:

- 2 Salmon fillets, 6 ounces (170gr) each
- 1 teaspoon olive oil
- Salt and ground black pepper, to taste
- Oil spray for greasing

Directions:

1. Mix all the listed ingredients for the dill sauce in a bowl. Drizzle the salmon fillet with oil and season accordingly with salt and pepper.
2. Line the bottom of the basket with foil and place the fillet in the basket, cooking it for 10 minutes at around 400° F (205°C), flipping halfway through. When done, shift it to a serving bowl and serve it with the side of sauce made earlier.

Per serving:

Calories 374 | Total Fat 11.4g 15% | Total Carbohydrate 14.5g 5% | Dietary Fiber 0.3g 1% | Protein 52.1g

― Cajun Scallops ―

Prep: 15 Minutes | Cook Time: 6 Minutes | Makes: 1 Serving

Ingredients:

- 10 Sea scallops
- salt, to taste
- 1 teaspoon of Cajun seasoning
- Cooking spray
- 1 tablespoon Garlic butter

Directions:

1. Start by seasoning scallops with salt and Cajun seasoning in a bowl.
2. Grease the inside of the air fryer with oil and arrange the scallops in them, cooking them for around 6 minutes at about 400 ° F (205°C). Serve with melted garlic butter.

Per serving:

Calories 358 | Total Fat 4.2g 5% | Total Carbohydrate 23.9g 9% | Dietary Fiber 0.3g 1% | Protein 52.8g

― Sweet Glazed Salmon ―

Prep: 15 Minutes | Cook Time: 12 Minutes | Makes: 2 Servings

Ingredients:

- 4 cup stevia
- ½ cup sweet soy sauce
- 2 ounces (60gr) of orange zest
- 2 tablespoons Lemon juice
- ½ tablespoon Red Wine Vinegar
- 2 teaspoons olive oil
- 4 cloves of garlic
- 1 scallion, chopped finely
- 2 salmon fillets, 4 ounces each
- oil spray for greasing
- Salt and black pepper

Directions:

1. Start by mixing stevia, soy sauce, orange zest, lemon juice, red wine vinegar, oil, and garlic minced in a saucepan and heat until it thickens.
2. Coat the fish with oil spray and season with salt and pepper. Then shift the fish in the thickened sauce and coat it.
3. Line the bottom of the basket of the air fryer with foil and place the coated fillet, cooking them at around 390 ° F (200°C) for about 10 to 12 minutes. Flip the fillet halfway in the cooking to ensure an even cook throughout.
4. Once cooked, glaze the fish with the additional sauce and serve with a topping of scallions.

Per serving:

Calories 355 | Total Fat 16.2g 21% | Total Carbohydrate 14.9g 5% | Dietary Fiber 3.9g 14% | Protein 39.6g

Sundried Tomato with Salmon

Prep: 15 Minutes | Cook Time: 10 Minutes | Makes: 2 Servings

Ingredients:

- 2 tablespoons Sun-Dried Tomato
- Salt and black pepper, to taste
- ¼ cup chopped fresh parsley
- 2 salmon fillets, 6 ounces (170gr) each
- Oil spray for greasing
- 4 Cherry tomatoes
- 1-½ cup broccoli

Directions:

1. Start by preheating the air fryer to around 350 ° F (180°C). Mix the sun-dried tomatoes, salt, and pepper in a bowl. Place the fish in the bowl and mix it with it. Grease both sides of the salmon with oil spray and place it in the bowl with sun-dried tomatoes, cherry tomatoes, and broccoli. Toss again with oil spray. Adjust salt and black pepper.

2. Add it to an air fryer basket lined with aluminum foil. Cook them for around 10 minutes at about 400 ° F (205°C). Make sure to flip the fillet halfway in the cooking. When done, shift everything to a serving bowl and serve.

Per serving:

Calories 315 | Total Fat 12.9g 17% | Total Carbohydrate 14.7g 5% | Dietary Fiber 4.8g 17% | Protein 38.5g

Frozen Fish Fillet with Mayonnaise

Prep: 15 Minutes | Cook Time: 18 Minutes | Makes: 2 Servings

Ingredients:

- 2-4 frozen salmon fillets, 6 ounces (170gr) each
- oil spray for greasing
- 1 cup mayonnaise

Directions:

1. Start by defrosting the fish and drizzling oil on both sides. Once coated with oil, shift it to the air fryer basket and cook it for around 18 minutes at 390 ° F (200°C). Make sure to flip it halfway through.

2. Work in batches according to the capacity of your air fryer. When done, shift the fish to a serving plate and serve with the side of mayonnaise.

Per serving:

Calories 821 | Total Fat 61.5g 79% | Total Carbohydrate 28.1g 10% | Dietary Fiber 0g 0% | Protein 41.1g

Smoked Salmon

Prep: 15 Minutes | Cook Time: 12 Minutes | Makes: 4 Servings

Mayo cream sauce:

- 2 teaspoons of fresh chives
- 6 ounces (170gr) of cream cheese
- 2 tablespoons mayonnaise
- Salt and black pepper, to taste
- ½ teaspoon of lemon zest

Fish ingredient:

- 2 salmon fillets, 6 ounces (170gr) each
- 3 tablespoons of olive oil
- salt and black pepper, to taste

Directions:

1. Mix chives, cheese, mayonnaise, salt, pepper, and lemon zest in a bowl. Drizzle olive oil over the fillet and season it with salt and pepper.

2. Once seasoned, shift the seasoned fillet into the air fryer and cook them for around 12 minutes at 390 ° F (200°C). Make sure to flip the fillet halfway while cooking. Once cooked, shift the salmon fillet to a serving plate and serve with the side of mayonnaise sauce made earlier.

Per serving:

Calories 770 | Total Fat 66.6g 85% | Total Carbohydrate 5.9g 2% | Dietary Fiber 0.1g 0% | Protein 41.1g

Pesto Salmon

Prep: 15 Minutes | Cook Time: 10 Minutes | Makes: 2 Servings

Ingredients:

- 2 salmon fillets
- 1 tablespoon of melted butter
- Salt and black pepper

Ingredients for Green Sauce:

- 6 tablespoons Greek yogurt
- Salt and black pepper, to taste
- 1 cup mayonnaise
- 1 teaspoon of pesto

Directions:

1. Start by coating the salmon with butter on all sides and seasoning it with salt and pepper. Mix the Greek yogurt, salt, pepper, mayo, and pesto in a bowl.

2. Place the salmon in the basket of the air fryer and cook it for around 12 minutes at 390 ° F (200°C), flipping it after 10 minutes and cooking it for another 10 minutes. When done, serve the fillet with a side of pesto sauce made earlier.

Per serving:

Calories 491 | Total Fat 31.6g 40% | Total Carbohydrate 20.2g 7% | Dietary Fiber 0g 0% | Protein 33.1g

— Salmon with Sauce —

Prep: 15 Minutes | Cook Time: 12 Minutes | Makes: 2 Servings

Sauce Ingredients:
- 1 teaspoon coriander seeds
- 1 teaspoon cumin seeds
- ½ cup packed mint leaves
- ¼ small pack of coriander
- 1 lemon (zest & juice)
- 2 garlic cloves
- ¼ teaspoon chili flakes
- salt, to taste
- 1/3 cup of water as needed

Salmon Ingredients:
- 1 lemon, juice only
- 2 salmon fillets
- salt and black pepper, to taste
- Oil spray for greasing

Directions:
1. Start by adding the ingredients for the sauce in a blender and blending them. Add a little water if it is too thick. Drizzle lemon juice on both sides of the salmon fillet and season it with salt and pepper. Mist salmon with oil spray.
2. Place the seasoned salmon fillet in the air fryer basket and cook it for around 12 minutes at 390 ° F (200°C), flipping it halfway through the cooking. When done, shift the fillet to a serving plate and serve with a side of sauce.

Per serving:

Calories 123 | Total Fat 5.8g 7% | Total Carbohydrate 0.8g 0% | Dietary Fiber 0.1g 0% | Protein 17.5g

— Coconut Cod Fillets —

Prep: 15 Minutes | Cook Time: 12 Minutes | Makes: 2 Servings

Ingredients:
- Salt and black pepper
- 1 cup of coconut milk
- 1 teaspoon of smoked paprika
- 1 pound (450gr) of codfish fillet

Directions:
1. Start by preheating the air fryer to 375°F (190°C).. Add salt, pepper, coconut milk, and paprika to a bowl and marinate the fish. Let the fish rest in the marinate for at least 2 to 3 hours.
2. Once it has marinated, shift it to the air fryer basket, and cook it for 12 minutes at around 375 ° F (190°C). When done, serve the fish on a serving plate.

Per serving:

Calories 518 | Total Fat 30.8g 39% | Total Carbohydrate 7.3g 3% | Dietary Fiber 3g 11 % | Protein 62.6g

Beer Battered White Fish Fillet

Prep: 12 Minutes | Cook Time: 12 Minutes | Makes: 2 Servings

Ingredients:
- 4 tablespoons arrowroot powder
- 2 tablespoons of Italian seasoning
- 1 teaspoon baking soda
- ¼ teaspoon of cayenne pepper
- 4 eggs, whisked
- 8 ounces (230gr) Plain yogurt
- 1 cup almond flour, Salt and black pepper, to taste
- ½ cup coconut flour
- 2 teaspoons smoked paprika
- 2 cod fillets, 6 ounces (170gr) each

Directions:
1. Mix arrowroot powder, salt, pepper, Italian seasoning, baking soda, and cayenne pepper in a bowl.
2. Crack and whisk together eggs and yogurt in a second bowl. Mix the almond flour, coconut flour, and smoked paprika in the third bowl. Add flour to arrowroot bowl and mix. Take the fish fillet, coat it with egg wash, and mix it with almond flour.
3. Line the bottom of the basket of the air fryer with parchment paper. Drizzle oil over the fish and place it in the air fryer basket, cooking it for around 12 minutes at about 390 ° F (200°C) When done, serve the fish.

Per serving:

Calories 488 | Total Fat 22.4g 29% | Total Carbohydrate 15.4g 6% | Dietary Fiber 2.8g 10% | Protein 55.8g

— Classic Catfish —

Prep: 15 Minutes | Cook Time: 8 Minutes | Makes: 2 Servings

Ingredients:
- 1-pound (450gr) catfish fillet
- ½ cup of coconut flour
- 2 teaspoons Cajun catfish fillet seasoning
- Cooking oil for greasing

Directions:
1. Start by cleaning the catfish and slicing it into a few pieces. Mix coconut flour and spice seasoning in a bag and add the catfish to the bowl, shaking the bowl to coat the fish evenly.
2. Grease the inside of the air fryer with oil, place the fish in the basket, and cook it for 8-12 minutes at around 400 ° F (205°C), flipping halfway through. When done, serve the fish.

Per serving:

Calories 823 | Total Fat 18.2g 23% | Total Carbohydrate 1.8g 1% | Dietary Fiber 0.8g 3% | Protein 159.6g

— Fish Fillet —

Prep: 25 Minutes | Cook Time: 12 Minutes | Makes: 2 Servings

Ingredients:

- salt and black pepper, to taste
- 4 tablespoons fresh parsley
- 2 cups pork rinds, grated
- 2 pounds (900gr) white fish fillet
- 2 eggs
- 1 cup almond flour

Ingredients for Sauce:

- ½ cup mayonnaise
- 1 tablespoon of drained capers, chopped
- 2 chopped jalapeños
- 1 tablespoon of lemon juice
- Pinch of chili flakes
- pinch of sea salt

Directions:

1. Start by preheating the air fryer to around 375 ° F (190°C). Mix the salt, pepper, parsley, and pork rinds in a bowl. Crack and whisk the eggs in another bowl. Add almond flour on a flat plate. Start by coating the fish fillet with almond flour, dip it in eggs, and finally give them a coat of pork rinds.
2. Once coated, arrange them in the air fryer basket in a single layer and cook them for around 12 minutes. While the fish is cooking, mix all the listed ingredients for the sauce in a bowl. Make sure to flip the fish halfway in the cooking to ensure even cooking.
3. When done, serve the fish with the side of sauce made earlier.

Per serving:

Calories 818 | Total Fat 47.6g 61% | Total Carbohydrate 9g 3% | Dietary Fiber 0.9g 3% | Protein 87.2g

— Simple Scallops —

Prep: 15 Minutes | Cook Time: 10 Minutes | Makes: 2 Servings

Ingredients:

- 8 sea scallops
- Salt and black pepper, to taste
- ¼ cup olive oil
- 2 tablespoons chopped parsley
- 2 teaspoons chopped capers
- 1 teaspoon lemon zest and juice
- ½ teaspoon chopped garlic

Directions:

1. Start by seasoning the scallops accordingly with salt and pepper. Grease the inside of the air fryer with oil

and arrange the scallops in a single layer, cooking them for around 6-8 minutes at about 400°F (205°C).

2. Meanwhile, mix parsley, capers, lemon zest, lemon juice, and garlic. Once the scallops are done, serve them with the sauce on top.

Per serving:

Calories 325 | Total Fat 26.2g 34% | Total Carbohydrate 3.5g 1% | Dietary Fiber 0.2g 1% | Protein 20.4g

— Fish and Okra Stew —

Prep: 25 Minutes | Cook Time: 25 -30 Minutes | Makes: 4 Servings

Ingredients:

- 2 fillets of tilapia fish, 6-8 ounces (200gr) each
- 2 tablespoons of olive oil
- salt and black pepper, to taste
- 2 teaspoons butter
- 2 teaspoons of almond flour
- 1 yellow onion, chopped
- 2 red tomatoes, cubed
- 2 green chilies, chopped
- 1 bunch of mustard leaves
- 2 teaspoons of Fish sauce, or to taste
- 2 cups sliced okra
- 2 cups fish stock

Directions:

1. Start by making small slits on both sides of the tilapia fish fillets. Drizzle oil over the fillets and season them with salt and pepper accordingly.
2. Place the seasoned fillet in the air fryer basket and cook them for 12 minutes at around 350 ° F (180°C), flipping halfway through. When done, take it out of the basket and let it cool down.
3. Meanwhile, take the cooking pot and melt butter in it. Cook almond flour for a few minutes until slightly brown, and then add onions, tomatoes, green chili, mustard leaves, fish sauce, and seasoning of salt and pepper. Next, add okra and let it simmer for 3 minutes. Now pour in the fish stock and let the boil come. Let it cook for 5 minutes, and add air-fried fish. Let it simmer for 5 more minutes until the stew is ready to be served. Enjoy.

Per serving:

Calories 296 | Total Fat 17.1g 22% | Total Carbohydrate 17.1g 6% | Dietary Fiber 3.3g 12% | Protein 20.1g

Crispy White Fish Fillets

Prep: 15 Minutes | Cook Time: 12 Minutes | Makes: 3 Servings

Ingredients:

- 2 organic eggs
- ½ cup coconut milk
- 2 cups seafood fry mix
- ½ cup pork rinds, grated
- 1 cup almond flour
- 1 teaspoon paprika
- salt and black pepper, to taste
- 1.5 pounds (680gr) of codfish fillets
- Oil spray for greasing

Directions:

1. Start by cracking eggs and coconut milk together in a bowl. On a plate, mix pork rinds and seafood fry mix. Add almond flour, paprika, salt, and pepper on another plate. Start by dipping the fish fillet in eggs and milk mixture, coat it with almond flour, and give it a coat of pork rinds.
2. For all the fish fillets, arrange them in a single layer inside the basket, cooking them for around 10-12 minutes at about 400°F (205°C). After about 10 minutes, flip the fish and cook it for the remaining time. When done, serve the fillet.

Per serving:

Calories 744| Total Fat 66 g 85% | Total Carbohydrate 3.4g 1% | Dietary Fiber 1.4g 5% | Protein 37.5g

Mahi with Brown Butter

Prep: 15 Minutes | Cook Time: 10 Minutes | Makes: 4 Servings

Ingredients:

- 4 Mahi fillets, 6 ounces (170gr) each
- Salt and black pepper, to taste
- Cooking spray
- ¼ cup butter

Directions:

1. Start by seasoning the fish fillets with salt and black pepper according to taste. Grease the fish, add it inside the air fryer basket with oil, and place it in the basket, cooking it for 12-14 minutes at 400 ° F (205°C), flipping the hallway through.
2. Meanwhile, melt butter in a pan and add garlic cloves. Simmer it for a few minutes and pour it over the fish.

Per serving:

Calories 193 | Total Fat 11.7g 15% | Total Carbohydrate 0g 0% | Dietary Fiber 0g 0% | Protein 21.1g

Salmon with Broccoli and Cheesy sauce

Prep: 15 minutes | cook time: 16 minutes | makes: 2servings

Ingredients:

- 2 fillets of salmon
- Salt and black pepper, to taste
- Avocado oil spray for greasing
- 1 cup of broccoli
- 1/3 cup of melted butter
- 1 cup of grated cheddar cheese
- ½ cup coconut milk
- ¼ teaspoon of garlic powder

Directions:

1. Start by seasoning the salmon fillet with salt and pepper. Then spray it with avocado oil. Add the broccoli to the basket of the air fryer and place the fish over it, cooking them for 10 minutes at around 390°F (200°C). Make sure to flip the fillet after 6 minutes.
2. Meanwhile, add butter and cheddar cheese in a saucepan and melt them. Mix it with coconut milk, garlic powder, and black pepper. Once the fish is done, serve it with a cheesy sauce.

Per serving:

Calories 839 | Total Fat 69.6g 89% | Total Carbohydrate 7.4g 3% | Dietary Fiber 2.6g 9% | Protein 48.8g

Salmon with Green Beans

Prep: 15 Minutes | Cook Time: 12 Minutes | Makes: 1 Serving

Ingredients:

- 2 tablespoons of olive oil
- 2 salmon fillets
- 2 teaspoons of smoked paprika
- Salt and black pepper, to taste
- 1 cup green beans
- Oil spray for greasing

Directions:

1. Start by drizzling oil over the salmon fillet and green beans. Then season them both with smoked paprika, salt, and pepper. Grease the inside of the air fryer with oil and add the green beans, followed by a salmon fillet.
2. Cook them for 12 minutes at around 370 ° F (190°C). Then flip the fish halfway. When done, shift everything to a serving plate and serve.

Per serving:

Calories 381 | Total Fat 25.6g 33% | Total Carbohydrate 5.1g 2% | Dietary Fiber 2.7g 10%| Protein 35.9g

Hearty Lemony Whitefish Fillet

Prep: 15 Minutes | Cook Time: 12 Minutes | Makes: 2 Servings

Ingredients:

- 2 tilapia fish fillets
- 1 teaspoon of onion powder
- ¼ teaspoon garlic powder
- 1/3 teaspoon lemon pepper seasoning
- 2 tablespoons of olive oil
- 1 lemon slices
- ¼ cup chopped parsley

Directions:

1. Start seasoning the fish fillet with onion powder, garlic powder, and lemon pepper. Then drizzle olive oil over the fillet and shift it to the air fryer basket.
2. Arrange lemon slices over the fillet and cook it for 12 minutes at around 390 ° F (200°C). When done, serve the fillet with a garnish of parsley.

Per serving:

Calories 380 | Total Fat 26.1g 33% | Total Carbohydrate 25.3g 9% | Dietary Fiber 1.5g 6% | Protein 12.5g

Breaded Razor Clams

Prep: 15 Minutes | Cook Time: 8-10 Minutes | Makes: 2 Servings

Ingredients:

- 6 razor clams
- 2 eggs, whisked
- 1 cup almond flour
- 1 teaspoon of garlic powder to taste
- 1 cup Pork rinds, Salt and black pepper, to taste
- ½ cup Parmesan cheese, shredded

Directions:

1. Start by washing the clams. Line the bottom of the basket of the air fryer with parchment paper. Crack and whisk eggs in a large bowl. Combine the almond flour, salt, black pepper, and garlic powder in another bowl.
2. Mix the pork rinds and parmesan cheese in the third bowl. Start by tossing clams in almond flour, dipping them in eggs, and coating them with pork rinds.
3. Place the clams in the freezer till they get hard.
4. Next, place them in the air fryer basket and cook them for around 8-10 minutes at about 390 ° F (200°C). When done, shift them to a serving plate and serve.

Per serving:

Calories 595 | Total Fat 38.8g 50% | Total Carbohydrate 6.5g 2% | Dietary Fiber 1.5g 5% | Protein 59.1g

Lemon Salmon

Prep: 15 Minutes | Cook Time: 10 Minutes | Makes: 2 Servings

Ingredients:

- ¼ teaspoon lemon zest
- 2 teaspoons of lemon juice
- 2 tablespoons olive oil
- ¼ teaspoon of turmeric
- ¼ teaspoon of cumin
- ½ teaspoon of red chili flakes
- 1/3 teaspoon of oregano
- Salt and black pepper, to taste
- 2 salmon fillets, 6 ounces (170gr) each

Directions:

1. Start by preheating the air fryer to around 350 ° F (180°C), and prepare the basket by lining it with foil. Mix all the listed ingredients in a bowl and coat the fish with them.
2. Once coated, place the fish in the air fryer basket and cook it for around 10-12 minutes at 400 ° F (205°C). When done, take it out and serve.

Per serving:

Calories 360 | Total Fat 25.2g 32% | Total Carbohydrate 0.7g 0% | Dietary Fiber 0.3g 1% | Protein 34.7g

Crispy Crab Claws

Prep: 15 Minutes | Cook Time: 15 Minutes | Makes: 2 Servings

Ingredients:

- 4 Crab claws
- ½ cup almond flour
- ½ cup pork rinds
- 2 whole eggs
- ½ cup shrimp paste, Cooking oil spray
- ½ cup of Chili-garlic sauce, as needed

Directions:

1. Start by cleaning the crab claws. Combine the almond flour and pork rinds in a medium bowl. Crack and whisk eggs in another bowl.
2. In another bowl, add shrimp paste and coat the crabs with the shrimp paste, followed by flour and pork rinds mix, then dip it in eggs and cover it with flour mix again.
3. Preheat the air fryer to around 400°F (200°C) for 6 minutes. Cook the claws in it for 15 minutes. When done, take the claws out and toss them with chili garlic sauce.

Per serving:

Calories 823 | Total Fat 18.2g 23% | Total Carbohydrate 1.8g 1% | Dietary Fiber 0.8g 3% | Protein 159.6g

— Tempura Fish —

Prep: 15 Minutes | Cook Time: 10 Minutes | Makes: 4 Servings

Tempura ingredients:

- 1 cup almond flour
- 1-1/3 cup arrowroot powder
- Salt, pinch
- Paprika, pinch
- 1 cup of water

Fish Ingredients:

- 12 ounces (340gr) codfish fillet
- 1 cup pork rinds

Directions:

1. Start by dicing the fish fillets into chunks. Add all the ingredients for the tempura batter in a bowl and mix them. Coat the fish first with tempura batter and then coat it with a layer of pork rinds
2. Once coated, place it in the air fryer basket lined with foil, and cook it for around 10 minutes at 400 ° F (205°C), making sure to flip it halfway through the cooking. When done, serve the fish.

Per serving:

Calories 336 | Total Fat 18.2g 23% | Total Carbohydrate 15.1g 5% | Dietary Fiber 0.8g 3% | Protein 26.6g

— Spicy Salmon —

Prep: 25 Minutes | Cook Time: 10 Minutes | Makes: 2 Servings

Ingredients:

- 2 fillets of salmon, 6 ounces (170gr) each
- 1/ 8 teaspoon cayenne pepper
- ¼teaspoon garlic powder
- 1/ 4 teaspoon onion powder
- ¼teaspoon oregano
- ¼teaspoon paprika
- 1 tablespoon olive oil
- salt and black pepper, to taste

Directions:

1. Start by preheating the air fryer to around 400 ° F (205°C). Add cayenne pepper, garlic powder, onion powder, oregano, paprika, and olive oil in a bowl and mix them.
2. Season the fish fillet on both sides with the spice mix and place it in the air fryer basket, cooking it for around 10 minutes. Cook the fish for 10 minutes at 400 ° F (205°C). When done, shift it to a serving plate and serve.

Per serving:

Calories 336 |Total Fat 19.1g 24% | Total Carbohydrate 0.8g 0% | Dietary Fiber 0.3g 1% | Protein 41.2g

— Mussels Dynamite —

Prep: 15 Minutes | Cook Time: 8 Minutes | Makes: 1 Serving

Sauce Ingredients:

- ½ teaspoon salt
- 2 teaspoons Sriracha
- 1 teaspoon stevia
- 2 tablespoons mayonnaise
- 6 tablespoons Parmesan cheese
- 2 teaspoons lime juice

Other Ingredients:

- 12 mussels

Directions:

1. Add all the ingredients listed for the sauce in a bowl and mix them. Pour the sauce over the mussels and cover them with foil.
2. Layer the aluminum foil inside the basket of the air fryer, and cook the mussels in it for 6-7 minutes at around 390°F (200°C). When done, take the mussels out of the basket and serve.

Per serving:

Calories 415 | Total Fat 25.1g 32% | Total Carbohydrate 11.1g 4% | Dietary Fiber 0g 0%| Protein 38.6g

— Fish Nuggets —

Prep: 12 Minutes | Cook Time: 8-10 Minutes | Makes: 4 Servings

Ingredients:

- ¼ teaspoon chipotle pepper
- ¼cup stevia
- 1 cup pork rinds, grated
- 2 large eggs
- 1 pound of salmon fillet
- Salt and black pepper, to taste
- Cooking oil for greasing

Directions:

1. Start by simmering chipotle pepper and stevia in a saucepan for a few minutes. Set it aside for further use. Crack and whisk the eggs in a bowl and add chipotle pepper and stevia. Whisk it well.
2. Preheat the air fryer to around 400 ° F (450gr). Season the salmon with salt and pepper. Coat the salmon first with egg mix and then with pork rinds.
3. Grease the inside of the air fryer with oil and place the nuggets in it, cooking them for 8-12 minutes, flipping halfway through. When done, serve the nuggets with a sauce of desire.

Per serving:

Calories 306 | Total Fat 17g 22% | Total Carbohydrate 0.2g 0% | Dietary Fiber 0g 0% | Protein 38.7g

— Crab Cheese Rolls —

Prep: 15 Minutes | Cook Time: 8-10 Minutes | Makes: 6 Servings

Ingredients:

- 6 ounces (170gr) of cream cheese, softened
- 1 cup crab meat
- 1 tablespoon garlic, minced
- 6 coconut wraps
- 2 tablespoons olive oil

Directions:

1. Start by mixing cream cheese, crab, and garlic. Arrange coconut wraps onto the flat surface and add a spoonful of the mixture in the center. Brush the edges with water and roll each of the wrappers. Then place them in the fridge and rest for at least 30 minutes.
2. Drizzle oil over the roll wrappers once rested in the fridge and arrange them in the air fryer basket lined with parchment paper, cooking them for around 8-10 minutes at about 375°F (190°C), flipping halfway through. When done, serve them.

Per serving:

Calories 282 | Total Fat 17.5g 22% | Total Carbohydrate 22g 8% | Dietary Fiber 1.5g 5% | Protein 8.7g

— Ginger Garlic Salmon —

Prep: 15 Minutes | Cook Time: 10 Minutes | Makes: 4 Servings

Ingredients:

- 4 salmon fillets, 6 ounces (170gr) each
- 4 finely chopped garlic cloves
- 1 tablespoon coconut amino
- 1-inch (25mm) finely chopped ginger
- Salt and black pepper, to taste
- ¼ teaspoon of Red chili flakes
- 4 tablespoons melted butter

Directions:

1. Start by preheating the air fryer to around 350 ° F (180°C), and line the bottom with foil. Place the fish in the prepared basket.
2. Mix garlic, coconut amino, ginger, salt, pepper, red chili flakes, and butter in a bowl and pour it over the salmon.
3. Cook the salmon in the air fryer basket lined with foil for around 10 minutes at 400°F (205°C), flipping halfway through. When done, shift it to a serving bowl and serve.

Per serving:

Calories 331 | Total Fat 22g 28% | Total Carbohydrate 1g 0% | Dietary Fiber 0.1g 0% | Protein 33.3g

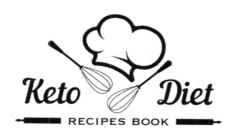

Chapter

10

Side Dishes and Vegetables

— Cheesy Spicy Cabbage —
Prep: 16 Minutes | Cook Time: 12-16 Minutes | Makes: 4 Servings

Ingredients:
- 2 pounds (900gr) of green cabbage
- 2 tablespoons olive oil
- ½ teaspoon salt
- ½ teaspoon ground pepper
- 1 teaspoon garlic powder
- 1 teaspoon onion powder
- 6 tablespoons grated Parmesan cheese

Directions:
1. Preheat the air fryer for 6 minutes at 350 ° F (180°C. Cut the cabbage into 2 inches wedges. Then coat the wedges with olive oil. Season the wedges with salt, pepper, garlic powder, onion powder, and parmesan cheese.
2. Work in batches or according to the capacity of the air fryer basket; arrange the wedges into a basket lined with parchment paper.
3. Air fries it at 375 ° F (190°C) for 12-16 minutes. Once browned from edges, take out and serve.

Per serving:

Calories 167 | Total Fat 10.3g 13% | Total Carbohydrate 14.8g 5% | Dietary Fiber 5.8g 21% | Protein 7.6g

— Cauliflower Biscuits —
Prep: 15 Minutes | Cook Time: 12-16 Minutes | Makes: 2 Servings

Ingredients:
- 1 .5 cups of cauliflower, florets
- 4 garlic cloves, minced
- 4 large eggs
- 1 cup shredded cheddar cheese
- ½ cup low-fat plain Greek yogurt
- ¼ cup diced scallions
- Salt and ground black pepper, to taste
- Oil spray for greasing

Directions:
1. First, preheat the air fryer before cooking at 400 ° F (205°C) for 4-6 minutes. Pulse the cauliflower into grainy consistency in a food processor. Then add garlic cloves, eggs, cheese, yogurt, scallion, salt, and pepper. Pulse it again and make a thick consistency.
2. Then divide this mixture into oil grease ramekins according to the material prepared.
3. Add the ramekins to the air fryer basket. Air fry at 350 ° F (180°C) for 12 -16 minutes. Once it's done, serve.

Per serving:

Calories 592 | Total Fat 29g 37% | Total Carbohydrate 19.7g 7% | Dietary Fiber 1.1g 4% | Protein 63.7g

— Cauliflower Rice —

Prep: 16 Minutes | Cook Time: 20 Minutes | Makes: 2 Servings

Ingredients:

- 12 ounces (340gr) cauliflower florets, frozen
- Oil spray for greasing
- 2 teaspoons soy sauce
- 2 teaspoons sesame oil
- 1 teaspoon garlic powder
- 1/3 cup frozen peas
- ¼ cup diced carrots
- Salt and black pepper, to taste

Directions:

1. Take the frozen cauliflower florets and add them to the blender. Pulse into grainy consistency. Then add it to the air fryer-safe bowl greased with oil spray. Add the bowl to a basket of the air fryer.
2. Add the basket to the unit. Airy it at 400°F (205°C) for 10 minutes.
3. Take out the basket and add soy sauce and sesame oil.
4. Stir the cauliflower rice and add garlic powder, then add reaming veggies.
5. Air fry again for 10 minutes at 400° F (205°C), stirring halfway through. Once it's done, serve with a seasoning of salt and black pepper.

Per serving:

Calories 119 | Total Fat 5.1g 6% | Total Carbohydrate 15.6g 6% | Dietary Fiber 6.3g 22% | Protein 5.4g

— Roast Celeriac —

Prep: 17 Minutes | Cook Time: 22 Minutes | Makes: 1 Serving

Ingredients:

- 1 cup celeriac, sliced
- 2 tablespoons olive oil
- Salt and black pepper
- 1 lemon, juice
- ¼ cup of fresh herbs

Directions:

1. Preheat the air fryer before cooking at 390 ° F (200°C) for a few minutes. Trim and cut the root of celeriac and slice it into strips. Then cut it into chunks. Add it to a large bowl with olive oil, salt, pepper, and lemon juice.
2. Layer the celeriac into the air fryer basket lined with parchment paper. Air fry it for 22 minutes at 390 ° F (200°C), shaking the basket halfway. Once done, serve with a topping of herbs.

Per serving:

Calories 327 | Total Fat 28.8g 37% | Total Carbohydrate 19.5g 7% | Dietary Fiber 6.2g 22% | Protein 3.6g

— Broccoli Fritters —

Prep: 18 Minutes | Cook Time: 12-15 Minutes | Makes: 4 Servings

Ingredients:

- 2 cups broccoli florets
- Salt and black pepper, to taste
- ½ cup superfine blanched almond flour
- 2 tablespoons nutritional yeast
- 1/3 teaspoon onion powder
- ½ teaspoon garlic powder
- ½ teaspoon smoked paprika
- 4 tablespoons unsweetened almond milk
- 2 eggs
- 4 green onions, sliced
- 1 cup of Sour cream

Directions:

1. Bring water to boil inside a pot and add broccoli to it. Cook the broccoli in it for a few minutes until softened. Drain and set it aside. Then dice it into smaller pieces. Add them to a bowl and season them with salt and pepper.
2. Then add almond flour, nutritional yeast, onion powder, garlic powder, smoked paprika, and almond milk. Then add eggs and green onions and make a fritter batter.
3. Put the dollops of batter onto an air fryer basket lined with parchment paper. Air fry for 12 to 15 minutes at 400 ° F (205°C), flipping it halfway through. Once all the fritters (cake/patties) are served with sour cream.

Per serving:

Calories 346 | Total Fat 27.1g 35% | Total Carbohydrate 18g 7% | Dietary Fiber 3.4g 12% | Protein 12.5g

— Squash Fries —

Prep: 17 Minutes | Cook Time: 22 Minutes | Makes: 4 Servings

Ingredients:

- 2 cups buttercup squash, and cut into sticks
- 2 tablespoons of melted lard, Salt, to taste

Directions:

1. Preheat the air fryer for 6 minutes at 375 ° F (190°C). Peel the buttercup squash, cut it in half, remove all the seeds, and cut it into French fries-style slices. Add it to a large bowl and toss it with melted lard and salt. Add it to an air fryer basket greased with oil spray. Air fry it at 390 ° F (200°C) for 22 minutes, shaking or tossing it halfway through. Serve once crispy. Enjoy.

Per serving:

Calories 105 | Total Fat 10g 13% | Total Carbohydrate 3.5g 1% | Dietary Fiber 0.5g 2% | Protein 0.6g

— Easy Popcorn —

Prep: 5 Minutes | Cook Time: 5-10 Minutes | Makes: 4 Servings

Ingredients:

- 1 cup corn kernels
- 1 teaspoon of avocado oil
- 1 tablespoon of butter
- Salt, a few pinches, or to taste

Directions:

1. Preheat the air fryer before cooking at 400 ° F (205°C). Take an air fryer basket and line it with foil in the shape of a round bowl. Add the popcorn kernels to a bowl and toss with oil.
2. Add it to the foil bowl and air fry at 400 ° F (205°C for 5-6 minutes, shaking the basket halfway. Collect un-popped kernels and add them to the air fryer basket to let them pop at 400 ° F (205°C for 5 minutes. Meanwhile, melt butter in a saucepan and toss popcorn with butter and salt. Enjoy.

Per serving:

Calories 52 | Total Fat 3.3g 4% | Total Carbohydrate 5.1g 2% | Dietary Fiber 0.3g 1% | Protein 0.5g

— Greek Roasted Vegetables —

Prep: 20 Minutes | Cook Time: 22 Minutes | Makes: 2-3 Servings

Ingredients:

- 1 rutabaga, peeled and sliced
- 1 eggplant, round cut
- 1 zucchini, rounds
- 1 red onion, circle
- 1 large tomato, rounds
- 1 cup of extra virgin olive oil
- 2 cloves garlic
- 2 teaspoons oregano
- Salt and black pepper, to taste
- 2 sprigs thyme

Topping Ingredients:

- 1 cup Feta cheese
- 1 cup olives

Directions:

1. Add rutabaga, eggplants, zucchini, onion, tomatoes, olive oil, garlic, oregano, salt, pepper, and thyme in a large bowl. Toss for fine mixing.
2. Add it to an air fryer basket lined with parchment paper. Air fry for 22 minutes at 390°F (200°C). Serve the veggies with toppings. Enjoy.

Per serving:

Calories 665 | Total Fat 62.7g 80% | Total Carbohydrate 25.2g 9% | Dietary Fiber 9.6g 34% | Protein 9.4g

— Vegetable Casserole —

Prep: 15 Minutes | Cook Time: 20-22 Minutes | Makes: 2 Servings

Ingredients:

- 1.5 pounds (680gr) of green beans, trimmed
- 1/3 cup of onion, diced
- 2 tablespoons of olive oil
- 4 tablespoons of almond flour
- ¾ cup vegetable broth
- ½ cup coconut milk
- Salt and black pepper, to taste
- 1 cup of mushrooms, diced
- 1/3 cup parmesan cheese

Directions:

1. Preheat the air fryer before cooking to 400 ° F (205°C) for 5 minutes. Take a; large cooking pot and bring water to a boil; add green beans. Let it simmer for 3 minutes, then take it out and pat dry with a paper towel. Meanwhile, use a wok or cooking pan to sauté onion in olive oil and add almond flour, broth, and coconut milk. Let it simmer for 5 minutes.
2. Season it with salt and pepper, and add mushrooms. Let it cook for 1 minute.
3. Add green beans and parmesan cheese to a basket of air fryers. Transfer the skillet mixture to an air fryer basket as well. Air fry it at 400 ° F (205°C) for 14 minutes. Once done, serve.

Per serving:

Calories 331 | Total Fat 24.3g 31% | Total Carbohydrate 21.6g 8% | Dietary Fiber 9.3g 33% | Protein 13.5g

— Cheesy Zoodles —

Prep: 17 Minutes | Cook Time: 20 Minutes | Makes: 2 Servings

Ingredients:

- 2 large zucchinis, spiralized
- ¼ teaspoon of salt
- 2 teaspoons of olive oil
- 1 cup parmesan cheese, grated

Directions:

1. Wash the zucchini and pat dry with a paper towel. Prepare zucchini noodles by spiral cut. Add a pinch of salt to the zucchini noodles and let them sit for 20 minutes. Then, remove as much salt as possible by squeezing.
2. Toss it with olive oil and add it to a basket of air fryers lined with parchment paper. Air fry it for 20 minutes at 420°F (215°C). Top with parmesan cheese and serve.

Per serving:

Calories 362 | Total Fat 23.2g 30% | Total Carbohydrate 13.8g 5% | Dietary Fiber 3.6g 13% | Protein 30.9g

Cabbage Wedges

Prep: 15 Minutes | Cook Time: 16-20 Minutes | Makes: 2 Servings

Ingredients:

- ½ cup water
- 12 ounces (340gr) small head of green cabbage
- 1 lemon, juice only
- 2 teaspoons Cajun seasoning
- Salt and black pepper, to taste

Directions:

1. Take an air fryer basket and add ½ cup of water, then preheat the air fryer to 350 ° F (180°C) for 4 minutes. Now take the whole cabbage and discard any loose or white parts from outside.
2. Now slice the cabbage in half and cut it into wedges about 4 equal sizes. Coat the wedges with lemon juice and rub them with Cajun seasoning. Season it with salt and black pepper as well.
3. Add the wedges to the basket of the air fryer. Air fry it at 350°F (180°C) for 16-20 minutes, flipping halfway through. Serve hot as a perfect side to your main course.

Per serving:

Calories 85 | Total Fat 0.3g 0% | Total Carbohydrate 19.8g 7% | Dietary Fiber 8.5g 30% | Protein 4.4g

Leek Rings

Prep: 10 Minutes | Cook Time: 6 Minutes | Makes: 2 Servings

Ingredients:

- 4 medium leeks cut into rings
- 1 cup yogurt
- ¾ cup almond flour
- ½ cup coconut flour
- 1 teaspoon of paprika
- Salt and black pepper, to taste
- Oil spray for greasing

Directions:

1. Remove the green parts of the leeks. Slice the leeks in rings. Add the leek rings to a large bowl. Soak the leeks in yogurt for 15 minutes, then dust them with almond flour, coconut flour, paprika, salt, and pepper. Toss it well.
2. Add it to an air fryer basket greased with oil spray. Add the basket to the unit. Close the unit. Air fry it at 350°F (180°C) for 6 minutes, shaking or tossing the basket halfway through. Once it's done, serve.

Per serving:

Calories 140 | Total Fat 4g 5% | Total Carbohydrate 19.4g 7% | Dietary Fiber 3g 11% | Protein 6.3g

Cheesy Sesame and Balsamic Vinegar Green Bean

Prep: 12 Minutes | Cook Time: 6 Minutes | Makes: 1 Serving

Ingredients:

- 1 cup of green beans
- 2 tablespoons of sesame oil
- Salt and black pepper, to taste
- 2 teaspoons of balsamic vinegar
- Oil spray for greasing

Toppings:

- 2 teaspoons of sesame seeds
- 6 tablespoons of parmesan cheese, grated

Directions:

1. Preheat the air fryer before cooking at 400 ° F (205°C) for 6 minutes. Take a bowl and add green beans to it. Toss the green beans with sesame oil, salt, pepper, and balsamic vinegar.
2. Add it to an air fryer basket greased with oil spray. Bake it at 400 ° F (205°C) for 4-6 minutes. Toss the veggies halfway through. Once it's done, take it out and serve by tossing it with sesame seeds and parmesan cheese.

Per serving:

Calories 496 | Total Fat 42.9g 55% | Total Carbohydrate 11.4g 4% | Dietary Fiber 4.5g 16% | Protein 21.1g

Avocados with Mayo Sauce

Prep: 15 Minutes | Cook Time: 16 Minutes | Makes: 2 Servings

Ingredients:

- 2 large ripe avocados, pitted, sliced, and cut lengthwise
- Avocado oil spray for greasing

Ingredient for the sauce:

- 1 cup mayonnaise
- 2 tablespoons Sriracha chili sauce
- 1 teaspoon lime zest, grated

Directions:

1. The first step is to preheat the air fryer to 400°F (205°C) for 5 minutes. Cut the avocados into slices and mist them with avocado oil. Place it inside the air fryer basket greased with oil spray.
2. Air fry it for 14-16 minutes at 400 ° F (205°C), tossing halfway through.
3. Meanwhile, whisk the mayonnaise, Sriracha sauce, and lime zest. Serve the avocado slices with the sauce.

Per serving:

Calories 537 | Total Fat 49g 63% | Total Carbohydrate 27.1g 10% | Dietary Fiber 10.2g 36% | Protein 3.4g

— Mixed Vegetables —

Prep: 14 Minutes | Cook Time: 10 Minutes | Makes: 2 Servings

Ingredients:

- ½ cup cauliflower
- ½ cup broccoli
- 1 cup zucchini cut into ½ inch
- 1 cup bell pepper
- 1 cup red onion

Seasoning Ingredients:

- 2 tablespoons olive oil
- 1 teaspoon garlic powder
- Salt and black pepper to taste

Directions:

1. Cut the vegetables into equal slices. Take a large bowl and add vegetables to it. Then add olive oil, garlic powder, salt, and black pepper.
2. Now, add it to the air fryer basket lined with parchment paper. Transfer the bowl mixture to the basket of the air fryer. Air fry it at 390°F (200°C) for 10 minutes. Shake the basket halfway through. Once it's done, serve.

Per serving:

Calories 190 | Total Fat 14.4g 19% | Total Carbohydrate 15.7g 6% | Dietary Fiber 4g 14% | Protein 3.3g

— Bacon Cabbage —

Prep: 15 Minutes | Cook Time: 14 Minutes | Makes: 2 Servings

Ingredients:

- 2 ice cubes
- ½ small head of cabbage, 12-14 ounces (370gr)
- 2 slices bacon
- 2 tablespoons olive oil
- Salt and black pepper, to taste

Directions:

1. First, preheat the air fryer before cooking at 370°F (190°C) for a few minutes. Add two ice cubes to the air fryer basket. Add the cabbage on top of the cubes.
2. Air fry for 7 minutes at 370 ° F (190°C). Take out the basket and add bacon and olive oil over the cabbage. Air fry for 7 minutes more.
3. Transfer the cabbage and bacon to a serving bowl and add dripping from the air fryer basket. Season it with salt and pepper.

Per serving:

Calories 268 | Total Fat 22.1g 28% | Total Carbohydrate 10.7g 4% | Dietary Fiber 4.5g 16% | Protein 9.3g

— Pine Nuts and Vegetables —

Prep: 15 Minutes | Cook Time: 8 Minutes | Makes: 2 Servings

Ingredients:

- 1 cup of green beans
- 1 cup pine nuts
- ½ teaspoon garlic powder
- Salt and black pepper, to taste
- 2 teaspoons of avocado oil

Directions:

1. Preheat the air fryer before cooking at 400°F (205°C) for 6 minutes. Toss all the listed ingredients in a large bowl. Line an air fryer basket with parchment paper. Air fry it for 8 minutes at 400°F (205°C), shaking the basket halfway through. Once it's cooked, serve and enjoy.

Per serving:

Calories 483 | Total Fat 47.2g 60% | Total Carbohydrate 13.6g 5% | Dietary Fiber 4.7g 17% | Protein 10.5g

Cabbage Fritters with Sour Cream

Prep: 15 Minutes | Cook Time: 6-8 Minutes | Makes: 2 Servings

Ingredients:

- 2 cups raw cabbage, finely shredded
- 1 medium carrot, finely chopped
- 2 eggs
- 1 tablespoon sour cream, some more
- 3-4 tablespoons almond flour
- 1 teaspoon salt or to taste
- ½ teaspoon pepper or to taste
- ½ teaspoon of baking soda
- 1 teaspoon Cajun seasoning
- 2 tablespoons Olive oil
- 1 cup sour cream to serve

Directions:

1. Preheat the air fryer before cooking to 390°F (200°C) for 6 minutes. Now remove the outer leaves of the cabbage. Shred the cabbage using a food processor. Then add carrots. Pulse it until it gets shredded. Add it to a bowl and add eggs, sour cream, almond flour, salt, pepper, baking soda, and Cajun seasoning.
2. Grease hands with olive oil and make small balls.
3. Arrange the balls in the air fryer basket lined with parchment paper, and air fry for 6-8 minutes at 400°F (205°C) Enjoy with a dollop of sour cream.

Per serving:

Calories 316 | Total Fat 26.7g 34% | Total Carbohydrate 12.3g 4% | Dietary Fiber 3g 11% | Protein 9.5g

— Buffalo Broccoli Bites —

Prep: 20 Minutes | Cook Time: 18 Minutes | Makes: 2 Servings

Ingredients:

- 1 cup almond flour
- 1/6 teaspoons salt
- 2 cups broccoli, cut into 1½-inch (40mm) florets
- 4 tablespoons melted butter
- ¼ cup cayenne pepper sauce, keto-based
- Salt, just a pinch

Directions:

1. Preheat the air fryer to 310 ° F (155°C) for 10 minutes. Add almond flour and salt in a large bowl and mix it well. Toss the broccoli in almond flour.
2. Transfer the broccoli to the basket of air fryer lined with parchment paper. Air-fry it at 350 ° F (180°C) for 15 minutes.
3. Meanwhile, take a saucepan and melt butter in it. Then add cayenne pepper, almond flour, and salt. Once the broccoli is ready, transfer it to the serving plate. Toss desired sauce over the broccoli and serve.

Per serving:

Calories 349 | Total Fat 32.2g 41% | Total Carbohydrate 15.2g 6% | Dietary Fiber 6.8g 24% | Protein 7.1g

— Veggies Casserole —

Prep: 20 Minutes | Cook Time: 20 Minutes | Makes: 3 Servings

Ingredients:

- 1 cup jicama, cubed
- 1 cup fresh sprouts
- 2 teaspoons extra virgin olive oil
- 2 tablespoons thyme
- Oil spray for greasing
- ½ medium white onions, Salt and black pepper
- 2 slices thick bacon, chopped into bits

Directions:

1. Peel the jicama and wash, and then cube it to ½ inches (12mm). Set it aside. Clean the sprouts as well. Add olive oil, salt, pepper, thyme, and olive oil to a bowl. Add to it sprouts and jicama.
2. Transfer all this to the air fryer basket greased with oil spray. Air fry it at 375 ° F for 10 minutes.
3. Meanwhile, chop the bacon into bits. Once 10 minutes of air frying, add the onions and bacon to the air fryer and air fry for 10 more minutes at 350°F (190°C).
4. For a crispier result, air fry for 7-8 more minutes. Once it's done, serve.

Per serving:

Calories 231 | Total Fat 6.8g 9% | Total Carbohydrate 26.7g 10% | Dietary Fiber 13.2g 47% | Protein 10g

— Bacon Brussels sprouts —

Prep: 20 Minutes | Cook Time: 16 Minutes | Makes: 2 Servings

Ingredients:

- 1 pound (450gr) Brussels sprouts
- Salt and pepper, to taste
- 1 tablespoon Olive Oil
- 1/3 cup of bacon bits

Directions:

1. Trim the bottom ends of the Brussels sprouts. Season it with salt, black pepper, and olive oil. Place it inside the air fryer basket greased with oil spray. Top it with bacon bits.
2. Air fry it for 8 minutes at 400 ° F (205°C). Take out the bacon bits after 8 minutes. Then again, air fry it for 8 minutes. Once it's done, serve.

Per serving:

Calories 466 | Total Fat 31.6g 40% | Total Carbohydrate 21.5g 8% | Dietary Fiber 8.5g 30% | Protein 28.9g

— Cauliflower Bites —

Prep: 16 Minutes | Cook Time: 20 Minutes | Makes: 4 Servings

Ingredients:

- 1 head cauliflower, florets
- ½ cup thick yogurt
- 1 tablespoon gram flour
- 1 tablespoon ginger garlic paste
- 1 teaspoon Garam Masala
- ½ teaspoon cayenne
- ½ teaspoon ground turmeric
- ½ tablespoon dried fenugreek leaves
- ½ teaspoon ground cumin
- ½ teaspoon carom seeds
- Oil spray for greasing
- Salt, to taste

Directions:

1. Cut the cauliflower into bite-size florets. Wash and pat dry with a paper towel. Take a bowl and add all the listed ingredients along with the cauliflower. Toss to coat the cauliflower well.
2. Add it to an air fryer basket lined with parchment paper. Air fry it at 350 ° F (180°C) for 22 minutes. Work in batches according to the capacity of the air fryer. Once done, serve with a drizzle of lemon juice on top. Enjoy.

Per serving:

Calories 53 | Total Fat 0.9g 1% | Total Carbohydrate 9.5g 3% | Dietary Fiber 2.3g 8% | Protein 2.9g

Asparagus Salad
with Feta Vinaigrette

Prep: 20 Minutes | Cook Time: 8 Minutes | Makes: 2 Servings

Ingredients:

- 1 pound (450gr) asparagus
- 2 tablespoons olive oil, divided
- Salt and pepper, to taste

Feta vinaigrette ingredients:

- 1 tablespoon balsamic vinegar
- 1 small shallot, finely chopped
- ¼cup fresh mint, finely chopped
- 6 ounces (170gr) feta, crumbled
- 4 tablespoons fresh dill, roughly chopped

Directions:

1. Preheat the air fryer before cooking to 355°F (180°C) for 8 minutes; toss the asparagus with oil, salt, and black pepper.
2. Air fry it by adding it to an air fryer basket lined with parchment paper for 8 minutes at 400 ° F (180°C).
3. Once done, add it to a serving plate. Mix vinegar, shallots, mint, feta, and dill separately. Toss it over the air-fried asparagus. Serve a delicious salad.

Per serving:

Calories 412 | Total Fat 32.7g 42% | Total Carbohydrate 16.8g 6% | Dietary Fiber 6.4g 23% | Protein 18.7g

— Spiced Cabbage —

Prep: 5 Minutes | Cook Time: 12 Minutes | Makes: 2 Servings

Ingredients:

- ½ head green cabbage
- 2 teaspoons apple cider vinegar
- 2 teaspoons olive oil
- Salt and black pepper
- 1 teaspoon garlic powder
- ½ teaspoon smoked paprika
- Oil spray for greasing

Directions:

1. Cut the cabbage in half, and then cut it into large quarters. Toss the quarters with apple cider, olive oil, salt, pepper, garlic powder, and smoked paprika, then add it to the air fryer basket greased with oil spray.
2. Air fry it at 400°F (205°C) for 12 minutes, flipping halfway through. Once done, serve. Keep an eye on the cabbage so the ends will not burn.

Per serving:

Calories 94 | Total Fat 5.2g 7% | Total Carbohydrate 11.8g 4% | Dietary Fiber 4.8g 17% | Protein 2.6g

— Tomato Soup —

Prep: 15 Minutes | Cook Time: 8 Minutes | Makes: 2 Servings

Ingredients:

- 2 cups tomatoes, puree in a blender
- 1 cup of coconut milk
- 4 basil leaves, whole leaves
- Salt and black pepper
- 1/3 cup parmesan cheese, grated

Directions:

1. Take a large heat-proof bowl that fits inside the air fryer basket. Add tomato puree, coconut milk, basil leaves, salt, and pepper to the bowl.
2. Stir it and add it to the air fryer basket. Close the unit.
3. Air fry it at 350°F for 8 minutes. Once done, transfer it to a serving bowl and garnish it with grated parmesan cheese.

Per serving:

Calories 366 | Total Fat 33.1g 42% | Total Carbohydrate 12.7g 5% | Dietary Fiber 4.7g 17% | Protein 9.8g

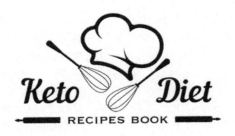

Chapter

11

Vegetarian Dishes

— Cheesy Baked Asparagus —

Prep: 10 Minutes | Cook Time: 22 Minutes | Makes: 4 Servings

Ingredients:

- 3/4 cup almond and cashew cream, unsweetened
- 4 cloves garlic, minced
- Salt and ground black pepper, to taste
- 1.5 pounds (680gr) of asparagus, stalks trimmed
- ½ cup plant-based Parmesan, grated
- 1 cup plant-based mozzarella
- Red pepper flakes, for garnish, optional

Directions:

1. Preheat the air fryer before cooking at 400°F (205°C) for a few minutes. Line a parchment paper to an air fryer basket. Grease parchment paper with oil spray as well. Add to the basket cashew cream and top it with garlic. Sprinkle salt and pepper on top. Then top it with asparagus.
2. Air fry it for 18 minutes at 350°F (180°C). Then add the topping of cheeses and air fry for 4-5 minutes. Then serve the cheesy air-fried asparagus. Enjoy with a sprinkle of red pepper flakes.

Per serving:

Calories 393 | Total Fat 2.9g 4% | Total Carbohydrate 27.7g 10% | Dietary Fiber 0.1g 0% | Protein 47g

Spinach Artichoke Stuffed Peppers

Prep: 20 Minutes | Cook Time: 12 Minutes | Makes: 6 Servings

Ingredients:

- 4-6 bell peppers, halved and seeded
- 1 tablespoon olive oil for drizzling
- Salt and black pepper, to taste
- 14 ounces (400gr) artichoke hearts, drained and chopped
- 12 ounces (340gr) spinach, thawed, well-drained, and chopped
- 1 cup almond and cashew cream, unsweetened
- 1 cup plant-based mozzarella cheese
- 2 cloves garlic, minced
- ½ cup of chopped fresh parsley for garnish

Directions:

1. Preheat the air fryer to 400 ° F (205°C) for a few minutes. Take an air fryer basket and line it with parchment paper. Cut the top of the bell pepper and scoop out all the seeds. Take a large bowl and add the remaining listed ingredients. Divide this mixture between the cavities of bell peppers.
2. Air fry it for 12-16 minutes at 360°F (180°C). Once it's done, serve.

Per serving:

Calories 106 | Total Fat 3.9g 5% | Total Carbohydrate 16.5g 6% | Dietary Fiber 6.4g 23% | Protein 5.1g

— Vegetable Mirepoix Bites —

Prep: 15 Minutes | Cook Time: 22 Minutes | Makes: 4 Servings

Ingredients:

- 4 celery stalks
- 2 carrots, peeled and chopped
- 2 onions, chopped
- Olive oil, as needed
- Salt and pepper, or according to taste
- ¼ cup coconut flour
- ¼ teaspoon garlic powder
- ½ teaspoon onion powder

Directions:

1. Take a bowl and add all the listed ingredients to it. Toss well for fine combination.
2. Transfer it to an air fryer basket lined with parchment paper. Air fry it for 22 minutes at 400 ° F (205°C). Once done, serve and enjoy.

Per serving:

Calories 46 | Total Fat 0.3g 0% | Total Carbohydrate 10.1g 4% | Dietary Fiber 2.9g 10% | Protein 1.4g

— Cheesy Cauliflower Bread —

Prep: 18 Minutes | Cook Time: 15 Minutes | Makes: 4 Servings

Ingredients:

- 1 large head of cauliflower
- 2 cloves garlic, minced
- 2 large eggs
- ½ teaspoon dried oregano
- 2-3 cups plant-based mozzarella shreds, plant-based
- ½ cup plant-based Parmesan, grated
- Salt and black pepper, to taste
- ¼ teaspoon crushed red pepper flakes
- ½ tablespoon freshly chopped parsley

Directions:

1. Preheat the air fryer to 400°F (205°C) for a few minutes. Grate the cauliflower in a food grater. Add it to a large bowl and add garlic, egg, oregano, 1 cup plant-based mozzarella cheese, plant-based parmesan cheese, salt, and pepper. Stir well, then transfer the dough to a loaf pan lined with butter paper. Add the loaf pan to the air fryer basket. Air fry it at 350°F (180°C) for 10 minutes.
2. Then, top it with the remaining mozzarella, crushed red pepper flakes, and parsley. Air fry it for 5 more minutes. Once done, serve and enjoy.

Per serving:

Calories 107 | |Total Fat 5.1g 7% | Total Carbohydrate 5.5g 2% | Dietary Fiber 1.5g 5% | Protein 8.5g

— Sweet Parsnip with Hazelnuts —

Prep: 15 Minutes | Cook Time: 8 -12 Minutes | Makes: 4 Servings

Ingredients:

- ½ pound (220gr) parsnip, trimmed, peeled, quartered lengthwise
- 2 ounces stevia
- 1 tablespoon olive oil
- 4 tablespoons hazelnuts, chopped

Directions:

1. Preheat the air fryer to 400°F (205°C). Take a bowl and toss the parsnip with stevia and oil. Add the quartered parsnip to the air fryer basket lined with parchment paper.
2. Air fry it for 8 minutes at 400°F (205°C). Top with hazelnuts and air fry for 3 minutes. Once it's done, serve.

Per serving:

Calories 145 | Total Fat 6.7g 9% | Total Carbohydrate 21.2g 8% | Dietary Fiber 6g 21% | Protein 2.1g

— Cauliflower Mac and Cheese —

Prep: 6 Minutes | Cook Time: 8 Minutes | Makes: 1 Serving

Ingredients:

- 1 head of cauliflower, cut into small florets
- 2 tablespoons of olive Oil
- 1 teaspoon of paprika
- 1/6 teaspoon of turmeric
- Salt and black pepper, to taste
- 2 tablespoons plant-based butter
- 3 tablespoons almond flour
- 2 cups coconut milk
- 1 teaspoon mustard powder
- 1 teaspoon hot sauce
- 2 cups plant-based cheese, mozzarella
- 2 tablespoons chopped chives, for garnish

Directions:

1. Coat the cauliflower florets with olive oil, smoked paprika, turmeric, salt, and black pepper. Add it to an air fryer basket lined with parchment paper. Air fry at 400°F (205°C) for 15 minutes.
2. Meanwhile, take a skillet and heat butter in it. Then add almond flour and cook for 1 minute. Then add coconut milk, mustard powder, hot sauce, salt, and pepper. Once thick, add cheese and add air-fried cauliflower to it. Serve and enjoy with chives.

Per serving:

Calories 428 | Total Fat 41.6g 53% | Total Carbohydrate 14.1g 5% | Dietary Fiber 6 21% | Protein 5.8g

— Roasted Edamame —

Prep: 16 Minutes | Cook Time: 12 Minutes | Makes: 4 Servings

Ingredients:
- 2 Cups Edamame or Frozen Edamame
- Garlic Salt, to taste
- Oil spray for greasing

Directions:
1. Take an air fryer basket and line it with parchment paper. Place the edamame in a bowl and toss it with garlic salt. Add the edamame to the air fryer basket and mist it with oil spray.
2. Air fry it at 400°F (205°C) for 12 minutes, shaking the basket halfway through. Once it's done, serve.

Per serving:

Calories 190 | Total Fat 8.8g 11% | Total Carbohydrate 14.2g 5% | Dietary Fiber 5.4g 19% | Protein 16.6g

— Pumpkin Schnitzel —

Prep: 14 Minutes | Cook Time: 24 Minutes | Makes: 6 Servings

Ingredients:
- 1 pound (450gr) turnip or swede, peeled and diced into 1-inch pieces
- 2 tablespoons olive oil, extra virgin
- 4 ounces (115gr) of plant-based cheddar cheese, grated, Salt and black pepper, to taste
- 2 tablespoons parsley, chopped
- 4 tablespoons hazelnuts, grated
- 6 ounces (170gr) of coconut flakes
- 4 eggs, whisked
- 1 pound (450gr) butternut pumpkin, peeled
- Lemon wedges for serving

Directions:
1. Simmer turnips in salted boiling water at a low flame. After 10 minutes, take them out. Drain and let it get dry. Add it to a bowl, season it with salt and pepper, and mash it into a puree. Preheat the air fryer to 350°F (180°C) for a few minutes.
2. Take a bowl and add cheddar cheese, parsley, hazelnut, and coconut flakes. In a medium bowl, whisk eggs and season them with salt and pepper. Slice the pumpkin into thick sticks, dip it in the eggs, and then into the cheese and coconut flakes mixture.
3. Add the pumpkin to the air fryer basket lined with parchment paper. Air fry it for 14 minutes at 400°F (205°C). Once it's done, serve it with mashed parsnips and lemon wedges.

Per serving:

Calories 318 | Total Fat 24.5g 31% | Total Carbohydrate 23.6g 9% | Dietary Fiber 6.5g 23% | Protein 7.3g

— Nutmeg and Coconut Scones —

Prep: 15 Minutes | Cook Time: 8 -16 Minutes | Makes: 6 Servings

Ingredients:
- 1 ½ cups coconut flour
- 2 teaspoons stevia
- 2 ounces (60gr) of plant-based butter, cold
- 1 egg, whisked
- ½ cup coconut milk

Toppings:
- ½ cup almonds, chopped
- ½ cup slivered almonds, toasted
- 2 tablespoons stevia
- ¼ teaspoon nutmeg, grounded

Directions:
1. Preheat the air fryer to 400°F (205°C). Take a bowl and add coconut flour and stevia. Add in the butter and rub it together. Now whisk eggs and add them to flour. Then add coconut milk. Knead it to form a dough.
2. Roll the prepared dough into rolls that easily fit inside the air fryer basket. Add the remaining topping ingredients in a bowl and top it over the rolls.
3. Add the rolls to an air fryer basket lined with parchment paper. Air fry it for 19 minutes at 400 ° F (205°C). Once done, serve and enjoy.

Per serving:

Calories 399 | Total Fat 28.6g 37% | Total Carbohydrate 26.5g 10% | Dietary Fiber 16.1g 58% | Protein 11g

— Crispy Tofu —

Prep: 14 Minutes | Cook Time: 16 Minutes | Makes: 2 Servings

Ingredients:
- 6 ounces (170gr) tofu, block extra-firm
- 6 tablespoons tamari sauce
- 4 teaspoons toasted sesame oil
- 4 teaspoons olive oil
- 4 clove garlic minced

Directions:
1. Drain and press the tofu using a tofu press for 10 minutes. Then cut the tofu into bite-size pieces. Add the tofu blocks to a bowl. Then add the remaining ingredients to a bowl and toss the tofu well. Let it marinate for 10 minutes at 400 ° F (205°C)
2. Then add the tofu in a single layer to a basket of air fryer lined with parchment paper. Air fry it for 16 minutes, shaking the basket halfway through. Once it's done, serve.

Per serving:

Calories 229 | Total Fat 22g 28% | Total Carbohydrate 3.4g 1% | Dietary Fiber 0.9g 3% | Protein 7.4g

— Cheese Sandwich —

Prep: 20 Minutes | Cook Time: 18-22 Minutes | Makes: 4 Servings

Bread Ingredients:

- 2 large eggs, whisked
- 2 tablespoons avocado oil
- 10 tablespoons almond flour
- 2 tablespoons of Psyllium husk powder
- 2 teaspoons baking soda
- Salt, to taste

Filling Ingredients:

- 2 tablespoons softened butter, vegan based
- 6-8 slices vegan smoked Gouda cheese

Directions:

1. First, prepare the bread; take a bowl and whisk eggs. Then add avocado oil and whisk again to combine. Add almond flour, Psyllium husk powder, baking soda, and salt in a separate bowl. Combine eggs with the flour mixture and stir well. If the batter seems too thick, add some water to it. Now oil sprays a loaf pan and pours batter into it.
2. Add it to the air fryer basket. Air fries it for 14 minutes at 320 ° F (160°C). Once done, take it out and let it sit for 10 minutes, then slice it. Butter one side of the bread slice and place the cheese slice on top of another. Make a sandwich and add it to the air fryer basket. Grease it with oil spray. Air fries it for 4 minutes at 350 ° F (180°C, flipping halfway through. Repeat it for the remaining slices as well. Once it's done, serve.

Per serving:

Calories 278 | Total Fat 23.1g 30% | Total Carbohydrate 14.8g 5% | Dietary Fiber 4.8g 17% | Protein 6.3g

— Garlic Chips —

Prep: 6 Minutes | Cook Time: 8 Minutes | Makes: 1 Serving

Ingredients:

- 10 cloves of garlic
- Pinch of salt
- 2 teaspoons of olive oil

Directions:

1. Slice the garlic into the thin cut. Toss it with salt and olive oil. Add it to an air fryer basket lined with parchment paper
2. Air fry it for 8 minutes at 380° F (195°C), tossing the basket halfway. Once done, serve. You can put the garlic on a paper towel to soak excess oil.

Per serving:

Calories 125 | Total Fat 9.5g 12% | Total Carbohydrate 9.9g 4% | Dietary Fiber 0.6g 2% | Protein 1.9g

— Avocado Chip —

Prep: 20 Minutes | Cook Time: 14 Minutes | Makes: 3 Servings

Ingredients:

- 3 large ripe avocados
- 1 cup plant-based cheese
- 1 teaspoon lemon juice
- 1 teaspoon garlic powder
- ½ teaspoon Italian seasoning
- Salt and black pepper, to taste

Directions:

1. Preheat the air fryer to 400°F (205°C) for a few minutes. Take a bowl and add avocadoes. Mash it with a fork and stir in cheese, lemon juice, garlic powder, Italian seasoning, salt, and pepper. Mix and mash everything well.
2. Now add a heaping tablespoon of mixture onto an air fryer basket lined with parchment paper. Air fry it for 14 minutes at 350°F (180°C). Once done, serve.

Per serving:

Calories 439 | Total Fat 41.1g 53% | Total Carbohydrate 19.5g 7% | Dietary Fiber 14.3g 51% | Protein 4.7g

— Easy Cheesy Chips —

Prep: 18 Minutes | Cook Time: 15 Minutes | Makes: 2 Servings

Ingredients:

- 2 cups plant-based mozzarella
- 1 cup almond flour
- Salt and ground black pepper to taste
- 1 teaspoon garlic powder
- 1 teaspoon chili powder

Directions:

1. Preheat the air fryer to 400°F (205°C) for 5 minutes. Take a bowl and melt mozzarella cheese in it by putting it into the microwave for 1 minute at high. Then stir and add the almond flour, salt, pepper, garlic powder, and chili powder.
2. Prepare dough and then knead the dough with your hands. Roll out in rectangles and use a knife to cut into triangles.
3. Spread it onto an air fryer basket lined with parchment paper. Air fry it for 15 minutes at 400 ° F (205°C). Once it's done, serve.

Per serving:

Calories 179 | Total Fat 13.2g 17% | Total Carbohydrate 11.7g 4% | Dietary Fiber 2.1g 7% | Protein 4.4g

— Cheesy Eggplant Parmesan —

Prep: 20 Minutes | Cook Time: 18 Minutes | Makes: 5 Servings

Ingredients:

- 2 eggplants, round cuts
- 2 teaspoons olive oil
- 1 cup tomato puree
- 4 garlic cloves, Salt and black pepper, to taste
- 1 teaspoon oregano
- 1 teaspoon avocado oil
- 1 -½ cups plant-based Parmesan
- ¼ cup fresh basil

Directions:

1. Preheat the air fryer before cooking at 400 ° F (205°C). Cut the top and bottom of the eggplant and then cut it into thin round slices. Season the round slices with salt and pepper. Then coat with olive oil.
2. Air fry by placing into an air fryer basket lined with parchment paper at 400 ° F (205°C). for 10 minutes.
3. Meanwhile, blend the tomato puree, garlic cloves, salt, pepper, oregano, and avocado oil in a blender. Remove the eggplants from the air fryer and top them with tomato puree and some mozzarella cheese.
4. Air fry for 5-8 more minutes at 400 ° F (205°C). Once the cheese melts, serve with a garnish of basil.

Per serving:

Calories 168 | Total Fat 2.5g 3% | Total Carbohydrate 23.2g 8% | Dietary Fiber 8.9g 32% | Protein 12.8g

— Zucchini Cheese —

Prep: 18 Minutes | Cook Time: 16-18 Minutes | Makes: 2 Servings

Ingredients:

- 2 cups of zucchini, grated
- 2 small organic eggs
- ½ cup plant-based cheese, grated
- 4 green onions, thinly sliced
- ¼cup almond flour
- Salt and ground black pepper

Directions:

1. Squeeze the zucchini and take out the moisture from it. Add it to the bowl and add zucchini, eggs, parmesan cheese, onion, and almond flour. Add seasoning of salt and black pepper.
2. Dump the pancake shapes of the mixture into an air fryer basket lined with parchment paper. Add the basket to the unit. Air fry for 16-18 minutes at 400 ° F (205°C)., flipping halfway. Once it's done, serve and enjoy.

Per serving:

Calories 59 | Total Fat 3.5g 4% | Total Carbohydrate 4g 1% | Dietary Fiber 1.5g 5% | Protein 3.9g

— Crispy Mushrooms —

Prep: 15 Minutes | Cook Time: 12-15 Minutes | Makes: 3 Servings

Ingredients:

- 2 cups oyster mushrooms
- 1 cup cashew milk
- 1 tablespoon lemon juice
- 1.5 cups of almond flour
- Salt and black pepper, to taste
- 1/3 teaspoon of garlic powder
- ½ teaspoon onion powder
- ¼ teaspoon smoked paprika
- ¼ teaspoon cumin

Directions:

1. Preheat the air fryer to 400 ° F (205°C). Wash and clean the mushrooms. Add mushrooms to bowl and pour in cashew milk and lemon juice. Let it sit for 30 minutes. Combine the remaining ingredients in a large bowl. Then take out the mushrooms and dip each mushroom into the almond flour mixture.
2. Add each mushroom onto an air fryer basket lined with parchment paper. Air fry mushrooms for 12-15 minutes at 400 ° F (205°C), flipping halfway. Once done, serve.

Per serving:

Calories 110 | Total Fat 7.8g 10% | Total Carbohydrate 6.8g 2% | Dietary Fiber 2.1g 8% | Protein 4.5g

— Easy Artichokes —

Prep: 15 Minutes | Cook Time: 16 Minutes | Makes: 2 Servings

Ingredients:

- 2 large Artichokes
- 2 tablespoons juice only
- 2 tablespoons olive oil
- salt and black pepper, to taste

Directions:

1. Preheat the air fryer to 400 ° F (205°C) for 2 minutes. Wash the artichokes and pat them dry with a paper towel. Remove the tips and short the stem, then cut it into length. Top it with lemon juice and oil, and season it with salt and black pepper.
2. Add it to an air fryer basket lined with parchment paper. Cook for 16 minutes at 320 ° F (160°C). Once it's crispy, serve it with a keto-based dipping sauce.

Per serving:

Calories 196 | Total Fat 14.2g 18% | Total Carbohydrate 17.1g 6% | Dietary Fiber 8.8g 31% |Protein 5.3g

— Simple Tomatoes —

Prep: 20 Minutes | Cook Time: 16 Minutes | Makes: 4 Servings

Ingredients:

- 2 tablespoons Olive oil
- 1 tablespoon Italian seasoning
- Salt and black pepper to taste
- 2 teaspoons balsamic vinegar
- 3-4 large tomatoes, round sliced

Directions:

1. Preheat the air fryer before cooking to 400 ° F (205°C) for a few minutes. Combine Oil, Italian season, salt, pepper, and vinegar in a bowl and dip each tomato slice for coating.
2. Then add the tomato slices to the air fryer basket lined with parchment paper. Air fry it for 12-16 minutes at 400 ° F (205°C). Once it's done, serve.

Per serving:

Calories 96 | Total Fat 8.3g 11% | Total Carbohydrate 5.7g 2% | Dietary Fiber 1.7g 6% | Protein 1.2g

— Veggies Rolls —

Prep: 15 Minutes | Cook Time: 16-22 Minutes| Makes: 6 Servings

Ingredients:

- 2 teaspoons of avocado oil for greasing
- ½ teaspoon grated ginger
- 2 garlic cloves, minced
- 4 ounces (115gr) of fresh shiitake, thinly sliced
- ½ cup shredded carrots
- ½ cup shredded cabbage
- ½ cup bean sprouts
- 1 tablespoon coconut aminos
- 1 tablespoon sesame oil
- 4 bulbs of scallions, thinly sliced
- Salt, to taste
- 12 coconut wraps

Directions:

1. Take a skillet and heat avocado oil in it. Then add ginger garlic and cook until aroma comes. Now add shiitake mushrooms and carrots and let it sauté for 5 minutes. Add beans, sprouts, coconut aminos, sesame oil, and scallions. Let it get cool, and season with salt. Mix it very well.
2. Place a coconut wrap on a flat surface and fill it, then roll to make a spring roll. Rub the edges with water before wrapping them to seal them.
3. Add it to an air fryer basket lined with parchment paper. Air fry it at 370 ° F (190°C) for 6-8 minutes. Once done, take out and serve.

Per serving:

Calories 118 | Total Fat 5.2g 7% | Total Carbohydrate 16.7g 6% | Dietary Fiber 2.4g 9% | Protein 1.6g

— Artichokes with Dijon —

Prep: 15 Minutes | Cook Time: 16 Minutes | Makes: 2 Servings

Ingredients:

- 10 cups of water
- Sea salt, to taste
- 4 whole artichokes
- 4 tablespoons of Dijon mustard
- ½ cup stevia
- 1/6 cup boiling water

Directions:

1. Boil water with a pinch of salt in a cooking pot. Turn off the flame. Then add artichokes to it and let it sit for 20 minutes. Drain and set aside for drying. Whisk Dijon mustard with stevia and add a few teaspoons of warm water. Baste the artichoke with it.
2. Add it to an air fryer basket lined with parchment paper, and air fry for 16 minutes at 360 ° F (180°C). Once it's done, serve.

Per serving:

Calories 70 | Total Fat 0.6g 1% | Total Carbohydrate 13.8g 5% | Dietary Fiber 7.5g 27% | Protein 4.7g

Cheesy Portobello Mushroom

Prep: 20 Minutes | Cook Time: 12 Minutes | Makes: 6 Servings

Ingredients:

- 6 Portobello mushrooms
- ½ cup tomato, pureed
- 4 garlic cloves
- 1 teaspoon dried thyme
- 4 teaspoons of vegan butter
- 6 tablespoons plant-based Parmesan grated

Directions:

1. Preheat the air fryer before cooking at 400 ° F (205°C). Wash and pat dry the mushrooms and cut the stems.
2. Meanwhile, blend the tomato puree, garlic cloves, thyme, and butter in a blender. Fill the cavity of the mushrooms with this combined mixture. Layer the mushrooms onto an air fryer basket lined with parchment paper, open side facing up.
3. Add the basket to the unit, and air fry for 8 minutes at 400 ° F (205°C). Take it out and top it with the equally divided cheese. Air fry for 4 more minutes. Once the cheese melts, serve.

Per serving:

Calories 88 | Total Fat 3.4g 4% | Total Carbohydrate 6.7g 2% | Dietary Fiber 2.1g 7% | Protein 6.2g

— Eggplant Bacon —

Prep: 22 Minutes | Cook Time: 15 Minutes | Makes: 4 Servings

Ingredients:

- 2 medium eggplants
- 4 tablespoons tamari sauce
- 4 teaspoons olive oil
- 4 tablespoons of stevia
- 1 teaspoon smoked paprika
- Salt and black pepper, to taste
- ¼ teaspoon garlic powder
- ¼ teaspoon cumin
- 1 teaspoon vegan Worcestershire sauce

Directions:

1. Preheat the air fryer to 400°F (205°C) for a few minutes. Wash and then pat dry the eggplants. Then cut the eggplants resembling bacon strips using a mandolin slicer. Take a small bowl and combine all remaining ingredients. Brush slices of eggplants with it.
2. Layer slices on to air fryer basket lined with parchment paper. Air fry it for 15 minutes at 400°F (205°C), flipping halfway. Cook until it turns into crispy slices. Serve!

Per serving:

Calories 111 | Total Fat 5.3g 7% | Total Carbohydrate 16.6g 6% | Dietary Fiber 9.9g 35% | Protein 2.8g

— Chocolate Pudding —

Prep: 15 Minutes | Cook Time: 6 Minutes | Makes: 4 Servings

Ingredients:

- ¼ cup of a dairy-free butter
- 4 tablespoons of stevia
- ¼ cup coconut milk
- 1 egg, whisked
- 1 cup of almond flour
- ½ cup of chocolate chips, melted
- Oil spray for greasing

Directions:

1. Combine the butter in a bowl and melt inside the microwave for 60 seconds. Then add stevia and coconut milk. Next, add the whisked egg and almond flour. Fold in the chocolate chips. Pour this mixture into ramekins greased with oil spray.
2. Put the ramekins in the air fryer basket. Air fry for 6 minutes at 200 ° F(95°C). Once it's done, serve and enjoy.

Per serving:

Calories 330 | Total Fat 28.5g 37% | Total Carbohydrate 16.3g 6% | Dietary Fiber 2.6g 9% | Protein 5.1g

— Candied Walnuts —

Prep: 20 Minutes | Cook Time: 14 Minutes | Makes: 4 Servings

Ingredients:

- 2 cups walnuts halved
- 6 teaspoons of plant-based butter, melted
- 2 teaspoons of vanilla extract
- 6 tablespoons stevia
- Cinnamon, pinch
- Salt, pinch

Directions:

1. Preheat the air fryer to 250°F (120°C) before cooking for a few minutes. Add walnuts to a bowl and add butter and vanilla extract. Then add stevia, cinnamon, and salt.
2. Toss and add it to an air fryer basket lined with parchment paper. Cook for 14 minutes at 200°F (95°C). Once cooked, serve, and enjoy.

Per serving:

Calories 177 | Total Fat 16.8g 21% | Total Carbohydrate 4.5g 2% | Dietary Fiber 1.4g 5% | Protein 2.5g

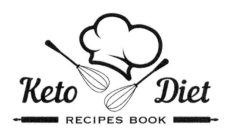

Chapter

12

Christmas Recipes

— Turkey breast —

Prep: 16 Minutes | Cook Time: 50-60 Minutes | Makes: 4 Servings

Ingredients:

- 1.5 pounds (680gr) of bone-in turkey breast
- 2 tablespoons olive oil
- sea salt and black pepper, to taste
- 1 tablespoon fresh rosemary, chopped
- 1 tablespoon fresh thyme, chopped
- 12 cloves garlic, peeled and chopped

Directions:

1. Start by preheating the air fryer to around 350 ° F (180°C). Pat dries the turkey using a kitchen towel. Drizzle olive oil all over the turkey and season it with salt, pepper, rosemary, and thyme.
2. Add whole garlic under the turkey's skin and shift it in the air fryer basket, cooking it for 25 minutes. After that, flip the turkey and cook it for another 25 to 30 minutes or till the skin becomes golden brown and the internal temperature reaches 165 ° F (75C). When done, remove the turkey from the air fryer and serve it.

Per serving:

Calories 306 | Total Fat 9.6g 12% | Total Carbohydrate 15.3g 6% | Dietary Fiber 1.1g 4% | Protein 36.2g

— Chocolate Cake —

Prep: 20 Minutes | Cook Time: 15-18 Minutes | Makes: 3 Servings

Ingredients:

- 1.5 cups almond flour
- 1 cup cocoa powder
- ½ cup butter
- 4 ounces (115gr) of cream cheese
- ¾ cup stevia
- 2 large eggs
- 2 teaspoons vanilla extract
- 1 teaspoon baking powder

Directions:

1. Mix the almond flour, cocoa powder, butter, and cream cheese in a bowl. In another bowl, blend butter and stevia using a handheld blender. Then mix eggs, vanilla, and baking soda, followed by the flour mixture.
2. Once mixed, pour the batter into a nonstick pan and add it to the air fryer basket, cooking it for 15 to 18 minutes at around 350 ° F (180°C).
3. Once cooked, take it out of the basket and let it cool down. Once cooled, flip it over and serve with a glaze of frosting chocolate.

Per serving:

Calories 604 | Total Fat 57.9g 74% | Total Carbohydrate 21.1g 8% | Dietary Fiber 10.1g 36% | Protein 15.6g

— Steak and Asparagus —

Prep: 10 Minutes | Cook Time: 16 Minutes | Makes: 2 Servings

Ingredients:

- 1 pound (450gr) sirloin steak, sliced
- Salt and black pepper, to taste
- 2 cups asparagus
- 4 tablespoons of olive oil
- 2 bell pepper, sliced
- 2 small onions, raw, chopped
- 4 cloves garlic, sliced
- ⅓ cup of soy sauce, or more to taste

Directions:

1. Start by preheating the air fryer to around 375 ° F (190°C). Season the steak with salt and pepper. Toss the asparagus with olive oil in a large bowl.
2. Arrange the asparagus into the r basket of the air fryer and cook them for 6 minutes at 375 ° F (190°C). Then take it out. Add steak, bell pepper, garlic, and onions to the air fryer and cook them for 8-10 minutes.
3. When done, shift everything to a serving bowl and serve them with keto soy sauce drizzle.

Per serving:

Calories 763 | Total Fat 42.7g 55% | Total Carbohydrate 22.8g 8% | Dietary Fiber 6.1g 22% | Protein 74.1g

— Whole Chicken Rotisserie —

Prep: 20 Minutes | Cook Time: 50 Minutes | Makes: 4 Servings

Ingredients:

- ½ tablespoon kosher salt
- ½ teaspoon freshly ground black Pepper
- 2 teaspoons garlic powder
- 1 teaspoon smoked paprika
- ½ teaspoon basil, dried
- ½ teaspoon oregano, dried
- ½ teaspoon d thyme, dried
- 4 tablespoons avocado oil
- 2 pounds (900gr) whole chicken, giblets removed

Directions:

1. Start by mixing all the listed spices with oil in a bowl and coating the chicken. Grease the inside of the air fryer with oil and arrange the chicken breast side in the basket, cooking it for 50 minutes at 360 ° F (180°C). then flip the chicken and cook it for another 10 minutes. Once its internal temperature reaches 165 ° F (75°C), take it out and serve.

Per serving:

Calories 457 | Total Fat 18.7g 24% | Total Carbohydrate 2.4g 1% | Dietary Fiber 1.1g 4% | Protein 66.2g

— Easy Duck —

Prep: 7 Minutes | Cook Time: 40-50 Minutes | Makes: 6 Servings

Ingredients:

- 2 tablespoons lemon juice
- 2 tablespoons olive oil
- 1 teaspoon minced garlic
- 1/6 teaspoon salt
- 1/6 teaspoon black pepper
- 3 pounds (1350gr) duck, clean and washed

Directions:

1. Start by mixing lemon juice, olive oil, garlic, salt, and black pepper in a large bowl, coating the duck by rubbing it all over it.
2. Arrange the duck in the basket of the air fryer and cook it for around 40 to 50 minutes at 300 ° F (150°C). Cook the duck till its internal temperature reaches about 170 ° F (75°C).
3. Once it reaches the desired temperature, remove it from the air fryer and shift it to a wire rack, letting it cool for 5 to 10 minutes before serving.

Per serving:

Calories 498 | Total Fat 30.1g 39% | Total Carbohydrate 0.3g 0% | Dietary Fiber 0.1g 0% | Protein 53.3g

— Roast Beef with Herb Crust —

Prep: 10 Minutes | Cook Time: 70 Minutes | Makes: 4 Servings

Ingredients:

- 2 teaspoons garlic powder
- 2 teaspoons onion salt
- 2 teaspoons parsley
- 2 teaspoons thyme
- 2 teaspoons basil
- ½ tablespoon salt
- 1 teaspoon pepper
- 2 tablespoons olive oil
- 2-pound (900gr) beef roast

Directions:

1. Start by preheating the air fryer to around 390°F (200°C) for at least 15 minutes before cooking. Mix garlic powder, onion salt, parsley, thyme, basil, salt, and pepper in a bowl. Drizzle olive oil all over the roast and sprinkle seasoning for a delicate coating.
2. Arrange the roast in the basket and cook it for 10 minutes at 400°F (205°C). After that, turn the roast, lower the heat to 360°F (180°C) and cook it for 60 minutes or till it reaches around 165°F (75°C).
3. When done, shift the roast to a wire rack and let it rest for 15 minutes before carving and serving.

Per serving:

Calories 489 | Total Fat 21.2g 27% | Total Carbohydrate 1.7g 1% | Dietary Fiber 0.5g 2% | Protein 69.2g

— Stuffing —

Prep: 20 Minutes | Cook Time: 6 Minutes | Makes: 4 Servings

Ingredients:

- 2 -3 cups pork rinds
- ¼ cup butter, melted
- 1 -½ cups chicken broth
- ½ cup celery, chopped
- ¼ cup onion, chopped about ½ small onion
- 1 teaspoon sage
- salt and black pepper, to taste

Directions:

1. Add pork rinds in a bowl, pour melted butter and broth over it, and mix it. Then add chopped celery, onions, and sage to the bowl and mix them in.
2. Shift everything to the air fryer basket and cook it for 6 minutes at around 320 ° F (160°C). Mix the stuffing halfway in the cooking to ensure even cooking. Season with salt and pepper and serve.

Per serving:

Calories 357 | Total Fat 26.9g 34% | Total Carbohydrate 1.4g 1% | Dietary Fiber 0.4g 2% | Protein 25.5g

Strawberries and Chocolate Chip Cookies

Prep: 20 Minutes | Cook Time: 7-8 Minutes | Makes: 6 Servings

Ingredients:

- ½ cup almond flour
- ½ teaspoon baking soda
- ½ cup butter salted, softened
- ½ cup stevia
- ½ teaspoon baking soda
- 1 egg
- 1 teaspoon vanilla extract
- ¾ cup strawberries
- ½ cup cocoa nibs

Directions:

1. Start by mixing almond flour and baking soda in a bowl. Add butter, stevia, and baking soda in a bowl and mix it using a handheld blender. Then whisk in eggs and vanilla extract.
2. Then add the flour mix to the egg bowl and whisk it using the blender. Fold in cocoa nibs and strawberries.
3. Line the baking tray bottom with foil or parchment paper, take a spoon full of the batter, and place it in the baking dish. Place the dish in the basket of the air fryer and cook it for 7 to 8 minutes at around 300 ° F (150°C). When done, serve the cookies.

Per serving:

Calories 292 | Total Fat 29.5g 38% | Total Carbohydrate 5g 2% | Dietary Fiber 2 7% | Protein 4.1g

— Glazed Ham —

Prep: 20 Minutes | Cook Time: 55 Minutes | Makes: 4 Servings

Ingredients:

- ½ cup lime juice
- 1 teaspoon of orange zest
- 2 teaspoons apple cider vinegar
- ⅓ cup stevia
- ½ teaspoon ground cinnamon
- 3 pounds (1350gr) of ham boneless, fully cooked

Directions:

1. Start by mixing lime juice, orange zest, vinegar, stevia, and cinnamon in a saucepan and heating over medium heat. Whisk the mixture occasionally till the stevia is completely melted and combined with the glaze.
2. Clean the ham and sore ½ inch criss-cross cuts on top of the ham. Arrange the ham in foil and brush half of the glaze over it.
3. Wrap the foil over the ham and place it in the air fryer basket, cooking it at 300 ° F (150°C) for 40 minutes. After that, open the foil and brush the ham with the remaining glaze. Close the foil and basket and cook it for another 5 minutes at 375 ° F (190°C).
4. Once done, shift the ham to a wire rack and let it rest for at least 10 minutes before serving.

Per serving:

Calories 371 | Total Fat 19.5g 25% | Total Carbohydrate 8.9g 3% | Dietary Fiber 3.1g 11% | Protein 37.7g

— Chicken and Bacon Kebab —

Prep: 10 Minutes | Cook Time: 12-14 Minutes | Makes: 2 Servings

Ingredients:

- 2 pounds (900gr) of chicken thigh fillets
- 8 ounces (230gr) of bacon
- 4 tablespoons of coconut oil
- Salt and black pepper, to taste
- 1 teaspoon of oregano, dried
- 2 teaspoons of garlic powder

Directions:

1. Start by slicing the chicken and bacon into 3-inch strips. Take the skewer and thread the chicken and bacon through it. Drizzle coconut oil over them and season them with salt, pepper, dried oregano, and garlic powder.
2. Arrange the skewers on a hot grill and cook them till they are cooked to desired tenderness, about 12-14 minutes at 375°F (190°C). When done, take them out and serve.

Per serving:

Calories 711 | Total Fat 49.4g 63% | Total Carbohydrate 2.1g 1% | Dietary Fiber 0.3g 1% |Protein 65.5g

— Crackling Chips —

Prep: 25 Minutes | Cook Time: 15 -30Minutes | Makes: 4 Servings

Ingredients:
- 2 pounds (900gr) of pork rind (crackling)
- 2 teaspoons of olive oil
- 2 teaspoons Bacon Flavored Seasoning, plus extra, to serve

Directions:
1. Start by slicing the pork rind into ½-inch thick strips. Line the bottom of a large baking tray with parchment paper and arrange the pork on top. Place the dish in the fridge and let it rest overnight. Then drizzle oil over the rind and season it with bacon seasoning.
2. Add half of the rind to the air fryer basket, drizzle some oil over and cook it for 10 to 15 minutes at around 390 ° F (200°C).
3. Once the skin begins to bubble, take it out and shift it to a bowl, season it with some more bacon seasoning, cook the other half and serve.

Per serving:

Calories 1316 | Total Fat 83.3g 107% | Total Carbohydrate 0g 0% | Dietary Fiber 0g 0% | Protein 145.8g

— Top Round Roast —

Prep: 20 Minutes | Cook Time: 50 Minutes | Makes: 4 Servings

Ingredients:
- 2 teaspoons of olive oil
- 3-4 pound (1700gr) beef top round, roast
- salt and black pepper, to taste
- 16 ounces (450gr) baby carrots
- ¼ cup beef broth

Directions:
1. Start by drizzling olive oil over the roast and season it with salt and pepper. Preheat the air fryer to around 400°F (205°C)
2. Arrange the roast in the basket (lined with foil) of the air fryer and cook it for 30 minutes at around 400°F (205°C)
3. Meanwhile, toss carrots with olive oil, salt, and pepper.
4. After 25 to 30 minutes, open the basket, flip the roast, and baste it with beef broth. Add the carrots and place them back in the air fryer, cooking it for another 18 to 20 minutes at 400°F (205°C). Take it out and let it rest for 10 minutes before serving.

Per serving:

Calories 753 | Total Fat 37.1g 48% | Total Carbohydrate 9.4g 3% | Dietary Fiber 3.3g 12% | Protein 89.9g

— Pork Roast —

Prep: 20 Minutes | Cook Time: 2 Hours | Makes: 8 Servings

Ingredients:
- 4 pounds (1800gr) of pork leg, boneless
- 4 tablespoons of olive oil
- 2 tablespoons garlic, granulated
- salt and black pepper, to taste
- 2 tablespoons of rosemary, dried
- 2 medium onions
- 4 medium button mushrooms
- 4 cloves garlic
- 2 teaspoons fennel seeds

Directions:
1. Start by preheating the air fryer to around 400 ° F (205°C). Clean the pork with water and dry it using a kitchen towel. Drizzle oil over the pork, rub it with garlic, and season with salt, pepper, and rosemary.
2. Slice the onions and mushrooms into thick slices and arrange them on a baking dish, greased with oil, in a single layer. Add garlic cloves and fennel seeds to the baking dish and arrange the pork over everything.
3. Place the dish in the air fryer basket and cook it for 40 minutes at around 430 ° F (220°C). After that, lower the heat to 355 ° F (180°C) and let it cook for at least 1 hour and 20 minutes. When done, take it out of the baking dish and serve it.

Per serving:

Calories 700 | Total Fat 47.2g 61% | Total Carbohydrate 4.4g 2% | Dietary Fiber 1.3g 5% |Protein 61.7g

— Simple Cake —

Prep: 22 Minutes | Cook Time: 25-30 Minutes | Makes: 2 Servings

Ingredients:
- 1 cup almond flour
- 1 cup almond milk
- ½ cup butter
- 4 large eggs

Directions:
1. Mix all the listed ingredients in a large bowl. Line the bottom of a baking dish with parchment paper and pour the batter into it.
2. Place the container inside the air fryer basket and air fry for 25 minutes at around 320 ° F (160°C).
3. To check whether the cake is cooked or not, insert a toothpick; if it is clean, the cake is cooked; if it comes out dirty, place it back in the air fryer and cook it for another 5 minutes. When done, take the cake out and let it rest on a wire rack before serving.

Per serving:

Calories 453 | Total Fat 45.3 g 59% | Total Carbohydrate 5.1g 2% | Dietary Fiber 2.1 g 7% |Protein 9.4 g

— Green Olives with Cheese —

Prep: 7 Minutes | Cook Time: 8 Minutes | Makes: 2 Servings

Ingredients:

- 4 large eggs
- 3/4 cup almond flour
- ½ teaspoon paprika
- ½ teaspoon garlic powder
- 12 ounces green olives
- 2 cups pork rinds
- Cooking spray (olive oil)
- 1 cup parmesan cheese, as needed
- Keto-based dipping sauce

Directions:

1. Crack and whisk together eggs in a bowl. Add almond flour, paprika, and garlic powder in another bowl and mix them. In the third bowl, add pork rinds. Remove the liquid from the olives, coat them with flour, dip them in eggs, and finally, give them a coating of pork rinds.
2. Grease the inside of the air fryer with oil and arrange the olives in them, cooking them for 5 minutes at around 400°F (205°C). After 5 minutes, flip the olives and cook them for 3 more minutes.
3. When done, shift them to a serving plate and serve them with a garnish of parmesan and a dipping side of choice.

Per serving:

Calories 549 | Total Fat 37.6g 48% | Total Carbohydrate 8.2g 3% | Dietary Fiber 2.8g 10% |Protein 48.9g

— Peanut Butter Cookies —

Prep: 20 Minutes | Cook Time: 8-12 Minutes | Makes: 4 Servings

Ingredients:

- 1 cup peanut butter, creamy
- 1 cup stevia
- 1 cup almond flour
- 1 egg, organic

Directions:

1. Start by mixing peanut butter, stevia, and eggs in a bowl. Line the bottom of the basket of the air fryer with parchment paper. Take a cookie scoop and scoop one big inside on the paper, and use a fork to make mash marks.
2. Add the basket to the air fryer basket and cook it for 8-12 minutes at around 400°F (205°C) or until golden brown. When done, take the cake out, and let it rest for 5 minutes before serving.

Per serving:

Calories 435 | Total Fat 37g 47% | Total Carbohydrate 14.3g 5% | Dietary Fiber 4.6g 16% | Protein 19g

— Turkey —

Prep: 10 Minutes | Cook Time: 30 Minutes | Makes: 4 Servings

Ingredients:

- 2 pounds (900gr) turkey
- 2 tablespoons of thyme, chopped fresh
- 1 tablespoon of sage, chopped fresh
- 1 tablespoon of rosemary, chopped fresh
- Salt and black pepper, to taste
- 3/4 cup of softened butter

Directions:

1. Start by cleaning the turkey and taking off the neck and giblets. Mix all other spices in a bowl. Gently let loose the skin on the turkey breast and legs to make pockets. Make sure not to tear up the skin.
2. Then dust the turkey with spice rub all over. Take the butter and spread it over the turkey.
3. Place it in a preheated air fryer basket lined with foil at around 350°F (180°C). Cook the turkey for 30 minutes at 350°F (180°C). Take the turkey out and let it rest for at least 15 minutes before serving.

Per serving:

Calories 679 | Sodium 395mg 17% | Total Carbohydrate 12.2g 4% | Dietary Fiber 4.9g 18% | Protein 78.3g

— Baked Cauliflower —

Prep: 15 Minutes | Cook Time: 40 Minutes | Makes: 2 Servings

Ingredients:

- 1 cauliflower, medium-sized
- 6 ounces of butter, salted
- 4 tablespoons of Dijon mustard
- 4 cloves of garlic, crushed
- 1 lemon, zest only
- Salt and black pepper, to taste
- 12 ounces of fresh parmesan
- 2 tablespoons of parsley, chopped

Directions:

1. Preheat the air fryer before cooking to 400°F (205°C) for 10 minutes. Take a saucepan and add butter to it. Melt the butter, add Dijon mustard, garlic, lemon zest, salt, and black pepper, and mix well. Whisk well and turn off the flame after 2 minutes. Brush it all over the cauliflower.
2. Air fry it for 30-40 minutes at 400°F (205°C). Baste halfway through with any remaining butter mixture.
3. Take it out and drizzle over the drippings from the tray. Serve with a garnish of grated parmesan cheese. Top with parsley and serve immediately.

Per serving:

Calories 547 | Total Fat 54.9g 70 % | Total Carbohydrate 10.8g 4% | Dietary Fiber 4.2g 15% | Protein 6.5g

Raspberry Glazed Chicken Drumsticks

Prep: 15 7Minutes | Cook Time: 2528 Minutes | Makes: 8 Servings

Ingredients:

- 8 skinless chicken drumsticks
- ½ teaspoon salt
- 1 teaspoon garlic powder
- ¼ teaspoon ground black pepper

Sauce Ingredients:

- 1 cup raspberry jam, unsweetened
- ½ teaspoon soy sauce
- ¼ teaspoon red chili flakes

Toppings:

- 2 tablespoons fresh parsley minced

Directions:

1. Start by pat drying the chicken using a kitchen towel and seasoning it with salt, garlic powder, and black pepper. Once seasoned, arrange them in the air fryer basket and cook them for 10 minutes at 380 ° F (195°C). Then flip the chicken and cook them for another 15 minutes.
2. While the chicken is cooking, start working on the glaze. Take a saucepan over medium heat and add jam, soy sauce, and red chili flakes. Bring it to a simmer for around 5 minutes or until it thickens slightly. Once thickened to desire, remove it from the heat.
3. When the chicken drumsticks are done, take them out and coat them with the glaze made earlier and place them back in the air fryer, cooking them for another 2 minutes. Once done, take them out of the basket and serve them with a sprinkle of parsley.

Per serving:

Calories 179 | Total Fat 2.6g 3% | Total Carbohydrate 26.3g 10% | Dietary Fiber 0.1g0% | Protein 12.9g

Peppermint Lava Cakes

Prep: 16 Minutes | Cook Time: 12-14 Minutes | Makes: 4 Servings

Ingredients:

- 2/3 cup chocolate chips, unsweetened
- ½ cup butter, cubed
- 1 cup stevia
- 2 large eggs
- 2 large egg yolks
- 1 teaspoon peppermint extract
- 6 tablespoons almond flour

Directions:

1. Start by preheating the air fryer to around 375 ° F (190°C). Add chocolate chips and butter to a microwavable bowl and place it in the oven, letting it melt for 30 seconds. Mix it till smooth, and then whisk in stevia, eggs, and egg yolk, and extract until thoroughly blended. Once mixed, add in almond flour and fold it over.
2. Grease the four ramekins with oil and dust flour over them, and pour the batter into each. Make sure not to overflow them and arrange them in the air fryer basket, cooking them for 12-14 minutes at 375 ° F (190°C) till their internal temperature reaches around 160 ° F (70°C).
3. When done, take them out of the basket and let them rest for 5 minutes to cool down.
4. Once cooled, loosen the cakes using a knife and run them around the edges. Take them out on a dessert plate and serve once cool by slicing.

Per serving:

Calories 456 | Total Fat 38.7g 50% | Total Carbohydrate 24.7g 9% | Dietary Fiber 2.1g 7% | Protein 4.9g

Crispy Turkey Legs

Prep: 20 Minutes | Cook Time: 40 Minutes | Makes: 4 Servings

Ingredients:

- ½ teaspoon smoked paprika
- 1 teaspoon seasoning salt
- 2 teaspoons garlic powder
- ½ teaspoon black pepper
- 1 teaspoon dried thyme
- 1 teaspoon Italian Seasoning
- 2 pounds (900gr) of turkey legs, rinsed and dried well with paper towels
- 6 tablespoons butter softened, salted, or unsalted

Directions:

1. Mix smoked paprika, seasoned salt, garlic powder, black pepper, thyme, and Italian seasoning in a bowl. Remove a tablespoon of butter and set it aside for basting and melt. Add butter to the spice mix and incorporate well. Pat dry the legs of the turkey entirely and coat it with herb butter, then apply the rub all over it.
2. Preheat the air fryer to around 400°F (205°C) 2 minutes before cooking and arrange the chicken in the air fryer basket, cooking it for 20-22 minutes at 400°F (205°C). After 20 minutes, flip the turkey, baste it with a tablespoon of butter, and cook it for another 20 minutes. Once the bird's internal temperature reaches 160 to 165 ° F, take it out and let it rest for at least 5 minutes before serving.

Per serving:

Calories 648 | Total Fat 41.6g 53% | Total Carbohydrate 2.1g 1% | Dietary Fiber 0.7g 2% | Protein 63.5g

— Filet Mignon —

Prep: 7 Minutes | Cook Time: 10 Minutes | Makes: 4 Servings

Meat Ingredients:

- 4 tablespoons Montreal seasoning
- ½ cup olive oil
- 4 filet mignon, 6 (170gr) ounces each

Blue Cheese Butter Ingredients:

- 1/3 cup blue cheese, crumbled
- 2 tablespoons parsley, freshly chopped
- ¼cup unsalted butter softened
- 2 garlic cloves, minced

Directions:

1. Mix Montreal seasoning and olive oil in a bowl and rub the steak with it, letting it rest for 10 to 15 minutes.
2. Meanwhile, mix blue cheese, parsley, butter, and garlic in a bowl and place it in the fridge. Preheat the air fryer to around 450 ° F (230°C) and place the steak in the basket lined with foil, cooking it for 6 minutes on one side, then flipping it and cooking it on the other for 4 minutes.
3. Once the internal temperature reaches around 135 ° F (55°C), remove the steak and shift it onto a plate. Add the prepared butter on top and let the steak rest for 2 minutes before serving. Enjoy.

Per serving:

Calories 516 | Total Fat 45.7g 59% | Total Carbohydrate 0.9g 0% | Dietary Fiber 0.1g 0% | Protein 27.1g

— Cottage Pie —

Prep: 16 Minutes | Cook Time: 35 Minutes | Makes: 4 Servings

Ingredients:

- 1.5 pounds (680gr) of cauliflower, cut into bite-size pieces
- 4 tablespoons of butter
- Pinch of paprika
- 4 egg yolks
- 4 garlic cloves, crushed
- 1 teaspoon of oregano, dried
- 2 small onions, chopped
- 2 sticks of celery
- 2.5 pounds (1150gr) of beef, ground
- 2 tablespoons of tomato paste
- ½ cup of beef stock
- 2 teaspoons of fresh thyme, Salt to taste
- 12 ounces (340gr) of green beans, chopped

Directions:

1. Start by filling two-thirds of the water in a saucepan and bringing it to a boil over heat. Once it begins to

boil, add cauliflower to the water and cook for at least 10 minutes or until it becomes soft and tender. Once it's cooked, drain out the water and shift the cauliflower back into the saucepan. Add butter, paprika, and salt to the saucepan and blend it using a stick blender till it forms a smooth paste. Next, mix in the egg yolks. Add all the other remaining ingredients mixed in the casserole dish.
2. Then add cauliflower on top casserole dish mixture.
3. Place the casserole dish in the air fryer basket and cook it for 25 minutes at around 350 ° F (180°C). When done, take the dish out and serve.

Per serving:

Calories 786 | Total Fat 34.3g 44% | Total Carbohydrate 23g 8% | Dietary Fiber 9.2g 33% | Protein 95.3g

— Almond Cookies —

Prep: 7 Minutes | Cook Time: 7-10 Minutes | Makes: 4 Servings

Ingredients:

- ½ teaspoon salt
- 2 cups almond flour
- 1 teaspoon baking soda
- 1 cup unsalted butter
- 1 cup stevia
- 2 large eggs
- 1-½ teaspoons vanilla extract
- 1/3 cup almonds, whole

Directions:

1. Start by mixing salt, flour, and baking soda in a bowl. Use a beater and beat butter in another bowl till it becomes creamy. Then mix in stevia and beat for 1 minute.
2. Then crack the eggs into the butter and add vanilla, mixing it with a hand beater till combined. Finally, add the almond flour mix to the bowl and beat at a lower speed till mixed. Place the dough in the fridge and rest for at least 6 minutes.
3. After that, take it out and roll it into small balls. Flat the balls with your hands. Arrange it onto an air fryer basket lined with butter paper, keeping the space between cookies. Top each cookie with one almond.
4. Air fry them for 7-10 minutes at around 375 ° F (190°C). When done, shift them to a cooling rack and let them cool before serving.

Per serving:

Calories 416 | Total Fat 41g 53% | Total Carbohydrate 7.6g 3% | Dietary Fiber 2.5g 9% | Protein 10.3g

— Cornish Hen —

Prep: 7 Minutes | Cook Time: 30 Minutes | Makes: 4 Servings

Ingredients:

- 1 teaspoon garlic powder
- 1 teaspoon onion powder
- 1 teaspoon paprika
- ½ teaspoon dry rosemary
- ½ teaspoon dry thyme, Salt and pepper to taste
- 2 pounds (900gr) of Cornish hen
- 2 tablespoons avocado oil

Directions:

1. Preheat the air fryer to 380 ° F (195°C) before cooking. Mix the garlic powder, onion powder, paprika, rosemary, and thyme. Coat the hen with olive oil, season with salt and pepper, and rub the spice mix made earlier.
2. Once appropriately seasoned, arrange it in the basket of the air fryer and cook it for 20 minutes at 390 ° F (200°C). Then turn the hen and cook it for another 10 minutes until the internal temperature reaches at least 165 ° F (75°C).
3. Once the hen reaches the desired temperature, shift it to a wire rack and let it rest for at least 10 minutes before serving and slicing.

Per serving:

Calories 320 | Total Fat 9.8g 13% | Total Carbohydrate 1.9g 1% | Dietary Fiber 0.7g 3% |Protein 53.2g

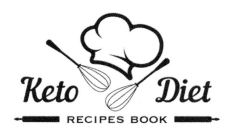

Chapter

13

Dessert Recipes

— Lime Macaroons —

Prep: 8 Minutes | Cook Time: 6 Minutes | Makes: 4 Servings

Ingredients:

- 4 large egg whites, room temperature
- 2/3 cup stevia
- 3 tablespoons gin
- 1, 5 teaspoons grated lime zest
- Pinch of salt
- ¼teaspoon almond extract
- 12 -14 ounces (370gr) of coconut, unsweetened and shredded
- ½ cup almond flour

Directions:

1. Preheat the air fryer before cooking to 400°F (205°C) or 5 minutes. Whisk egg whites, stevia, gin, lime zest, salt, and almond extract in a large bowl.
2. Then take a separate bowl and add coconut and almond flour and add to the egg mixture. Fold it well.
3. Dump the heaping tablespoon onto an air fryer basket lined with parchment paper. Air fry it for 6 minutes at 400 ° F (205°C). Work in batches. Once done, serve and enjoy.

Per serving:

Calories 367 | Total Fat 30.3g 39% | Total Carbohydrate 14g 5% | Dietary Fiber 8.1g 29% | Protein 7.3g

— Pine Nut Cookies —

Prep: 15 Minutes | Cook Time: 7-8 Minutes | Makes: 4 Servings

Ingredients:

- ¾ cup unsalted butter
- 1 cup stevia
- 3-5 large eggs
- 2.5 cups almond flour
- 1 cup pine nuts, chopped
- 1 teaspoon baking soda, or as needed
- 2-3 cups coconut flakes

Directions:

1. Combine butter and stevia in a bowl and mix using a hand beater. Then add eggs and again mix using a hand beater. Next, add almond flour and pine nuts. Once it's smooth, add the baking soda. Fold everything well.
2. Make the small dough and roll each dough into coconut flakes. Shape into cookies.
3. Arrange it onto an air fryer basket lined with parchment paper. Air fry at 320°F (160°C) for 7-8 minutes. Work in batches according to the capacity of the air fryer basket. Once done, set it aside and let it cool, then serve.

Per serving:

Calories 776 | Total Fat 79.9g 102% | Total Carbohydrate 14.3g 5% | Dietary Fiber 6.7g 24% |Protein 10.1g

— Coconut Meringues —

Prep: 12 Minutes | Cook Time: 5 Minutes | Makes: 2 Servings

Ingredients:

- 4 egg whites
- Salt, to taste
- ½ teaspoon coconut extract
- ½ cup stevia
- ¼ teaspoon cream of tartar

Directions:

1. Take a mixer and add egg whites. Attach paddles to the mixer to whisk until a stiff peak forms on top. Then add salt, coconut extract, and cream of tartar and mix. Gradually add stevia while keep mixing it at a low speed.
2. Then a layer of parchment paper inside the air fryer basket. Then pipe the mixture onto the air fryer basket. Air fry at 350°F (180°C) for 5 minutes. Then air fry at 250°F (120°C) for 10 minutes. Once it is cooked, let it cool, and serve.

Per serving:

Calories 38 | Total Fat 0.1g 0% | Total Carbohydrate 0.8g 0% | Dietary Fiber 0g 0% | Protein 7.2g

— Cocoa Cupcake —

Prep: 16 Minutes | Cook Time: 12-15 Minutes | Makes: 4 Servings

Ingredients:

- 2-4 small organic eggs
- ½ cup stevia
- 2 tablespoons of almond milk
- ¼ cup plain unsalted butter
- 1 teaspoon pure vanilla extract
- 1 -½ cups almond flour
- 1/3 cup cocoa powder
- ½ teaspoon baking soda
- Salt, to taste

Directions:

1. Combine the eggs and the stevia in a large bowl and whisk it well. Then, mix the almond milk, butter, and vanilla extract.
2. In a separate bowl, add all the listed dry ingredients and stir. Combine dry ingredients with wet ones and then mix for good incorporation.
3. Place the ramekins lined with muffin cups in the air fryer basket and pour the mixture into the cups. Air fry it for 12-15 minutes at 300 ° F (150°C). Serve and enjoy the cupcakes.

Per serving:

Calories 238 | Total Fat 23.8g 31% | Total Carbohydrate 5.7g 2% | Dietary Fiber 3g 11% | Protein 5.4g

— Vanilla Meringues —

Prep: 10 Minutes | Cook Time: 5 Minutes | Makes: 1 Serving

Ingredients:

- ¼ teaspoon cream of tartar
- Salt, to taste
- 4 egg whites
- ½ cup stevia
- ½ teaspoon vanilla bean extract

Directions:

1. Take a bowl and add egg whites to it. Use a hand beater to whisk until stiff peak forms on top. Then add salt, vanilla extract, and cream of tartar and again mix. Gradually add the stevia while mixing.
2. Then a layer of parchment paper inside the air fryer basket. Then pipe the mixture onto the air fryer basket. Air fry at 350°F (180°C) for 5 minutes. Then air fry at 250°F (120°C) for 10 minutes. Once it is cooked, let it cool, and serve.

Per serving:

Calories 35 | Total Fat 0.1g 0% | Total Carbohydrate 0.7g 0% | Dietary Fiber 0g 0% | Protein 7.2g

— Chocolate Chip Cookies —

Prep: 16 Minutes | Cook Time: 8 Minutes | Makes: 8 Servings

Ingredients:

- 2.5 cups almond flour
- ½ cup coconut flour
- Pinch of salt
- ½ cup unsalted butter softened
- ½ cup stevia sweetener
- 2 eggs
- 1 teaspoon vanilla extract

Add on:

- 1 cup chocolate chips, keto-based

Directions:

1. Preheat the air fryer before cooking at 350°F (180°C) for 5 minutes. Put all the dry ingredients in a large bowl. Add and whisk all the wet ingredients into a separate bowl
2. Combine the components of both bowls. Fold in chocolate chips at the end. Make small dough balls and place them on an air fryer basket lined with parchment paper, pressing down the balls to flatten them up.
3. Air fry at 350°F (180°C) for 8 minutes. Then transfer the cookies to a cool rack. Once it's cool, serve.

Per serving:

Calories 379 | Total Fat 34.3g 44% | Total Carbohydrate 15g 5% | Dietary Fiber 2 7% | Protein 4.5g

⸺ Lime Meringues ⸺

Prep: 7 Minutes | Cook Time: 15 Minutes | Makes: 4 Servings

Ingredients:

- 4 eggs, whites only
- Salt, pinch
- ½ teaspoon lime extract
- ¼ teaspoon cream of tartar
- ½ cup stevia

Directions:

1. Take a bowl and add egg whites to it. Use a hand beater to whisk until a stiff peak forms on top. Then add salt, lime extract, and cream of tartar, and again mix. Then add stevia and keep mixing using a hand beater. Then a layer of parchment paper inside the air fryer basket.
2. Then pipe the mixture onto the air fryer basket. Air fry it at 350° F (180°C) for 5 minutes. Then air fry at 250°F (120°C) for 10 minutes. Once it is cooked, let it cool, and serve.

Per serving:

Calories 63 | Total Fat 4.4g 6% | Total Carbohydrate 0.5g 0% | Dietary Fiber 0g 0%| Protein 5.5g

⸺ Eggless Cake ⸺

Prep: 22 Minutes | Cook Time: 12 Minutes | Makes: 4 Servings

Dry Ingredients:

- 2/3 cup of almond flour
- 4 tablespoons stevia
- 3 tablespoons of cocoa powder
- 3/8 teaspoon of baking soda

Wet Ingredients:

- ½ teaspoon of vanilla extract
- 5 tablespoons of coconut milk
- 2 tablespoons of olive oil
- 2 teaspoons of warm water
- Oil spray for greasing

Directions:

1. Preheat the air fryer before cooking at 350°F (180°C) for 5 minutes. Combine all the dry ingredients in a large bowl. In a separate bowl and add all the remaining wet ingredients.
2. Mix the dry ingredients with all the wet ingredients. Dump the prepared cake batter into a pan lined with butter paper and grease with oil spray.
3. Place the cake pan in the basket and cook for 12 minutes at 350 ° F (180°C). Check if the cake is made by sticking a toothpick in it. Let it shift to a cooling rack, and let it cool before serving.

Per serving:

Calories 142 | Total Fat 14.5g 19% | Total Carbohydrate 4.3g 2% | Dietary Fiber 2.1g 8% | Protein 2.2g

⸺ Simple Chocolate Pudding ⸺

Prep: 10 Minutes | Cook Time: 6 Minutes | Makes: 2 Servings

Ingredients:

- Oil spray for greasing
- 2 teaspoons butter
- 4 tablespoons dark chocolate
- 4 tablespoons of almond flour
- 6 ounces (170gr) of cream cheese
- 2 teaspoons dark chocolate, melted

Directions:

1. Take two ramekins and grease them with oil spray. Combine butter and dark chocolate in a bowl and microwave for 1 minute to melt. Then stir it with almond flour to combine. Pour this mixture into the ramekins.
2. And use a head beater to beat the cream cheese with chocolate syrup. Pour it over ramekins
3. Add ramekins to the air fryer basket. Air fry for 6 minutes at 375°F (190°C). Once it's done, serve.

Per serving:

Calories 483 | Total Fat 41.8g 54% | Total Carbohydrate 19.6g 7% | Dietary Fiber 1.3g 4% | Protein 9g

⸺ Chocolate Cheesecake ⸺

Prep: 10 Minutes | Cook Time: 10 Minutes | Makes: 4 Servings

Ingredients:

- 16 ounces (450gr) of cream cheese
- 1 cup stevia
- 2 eggs, organic
- ½ teaspoon vanilla extract
- ¼ cup unsweetened cocoa nibs
- Oil spray for greasing

Directions:

1. Take a hand beater and combine well cream cheese with stevia using a large bowl. Then add eggs and vanilla and mix unit frothy. Now fold in cocoa nibs. Take a spring form pan that easily fits inside the air fryer basket
2. Grease the spring form pan with oil spray. And add the mixture to it.
3. Add the spring form pan into the air fryer basket. And air fry at 300°F (150°C) for 10 minutes. Refrigerator for 2-4 hours before sourcing.

Per serving:

Calories 594 | Total Fat 51.7g 66% | Total Carbohydrate 19.4g 7% | Dietary Fiber 2.7g 10% | Protein 10.6g

— Peanut Butter Cupcake —

Prep: 16 Minutes | Cook Time: 12-15 Minutes | Makes: 4 Servings

Ingredients:

- 2 small organic eggs
- 2 tablespoons of stevia
- 1/3 cup peanut butter
- ¼ cup butter
- 1 cup almond flour
- ½ teaspoon baking soda
- Salt, to taste

Directions:

1. Combine the eggs and the stevia in a large bowl and whisk it well. Then pour in the peanut butter and butter, and mix again. In a separate bowl, add all the listed dry ingredients and stir.
2. Combine dry ingredients with wet ones and then mix for good incorporation.
3. Place the ramekins lined with muffin cups in the air fryer basket and pour the mixture into the cups.
4. Air fry it for 12-15 minutes at 300°F (150°C). Serve and enjoy the cupcakes.

Per serving:

Calories 406 | Total Fat 34.1g 44% | Total Carbohydrate 12.5g 5% | Dietary Fiber 4.4g 16% | Protein 19.2g

— Chocolate Chip Cookies —

Prep: 10 Minutes | Cook Time: 8 Minutes | Makes: 4 Servings

Ingredients:

- 1.5 cups almond flour
- ½ teaspoon salt
- ½ teaspoon baking soda
- 1-2 large eggs
- ¼ cup stevia
- 1 teaspoon vanilla extract
- ½ cup unsalted butter softened
- 1 cup cocoa nibs

Directions:

1. Preheat the air fryer before cooking to 350°F (180°C) for a few minutes. Combine the almond flour, salt, and baking soda in a bowl. In a separate bowl, whisk eggs and add stevia and vanilla extract along with butter
2. Now add dry ingredients to the wet ingredients and fold in nibs. Stir twice, and scoop the cookies onto the basket of air fryer that is lined with parchment paper. Air fry it at 325 ° F (160°C) for 8-10 minutes. Transfer to a cooling rack, and then serve.

Per serving:

Calories 305 | Total Fat 26.4g 34% | Total Carbohydrate 11.3g 4% | Dietary Fiber 4.7g 17% | Protein 12.3g

— 3 Ingredients Cookies —

Prep: 20 Minutes | Cook Time: 6 -8Minutes | Makes: 2 Servings

Ingredients:

- 1/3 cup peanut butter
- 1 egg
- 1 cup almond flour
- ¼ cup cocoa nibs, unsweetened

Directions:

1. Mix the peanut butter and egg in a bowl using a hand mixer. Then add the almond flour and incorporate the ingredients well. Refrigerate it for 10 minutes.
2. Make small balls out of the dough. Then press it down to make it flat, and top it with some cocoa nibs.
3. Add it to an air fryer basket lined with parchment paper. Air fryer for 6-8 minutes at 350°F (180°C).
4. Once the cookies are baked, take cookies out and let them cool on a wire rack. Serve and enjoy.

Per serving:

Calories 383 | Total Fat 32.7g 42% | Total Carbohydrate 12.6g 5% | Dietary Fiber 4.6g 16% | Protein 16.9g

— Pumpkin Bread —

Prep: 15 Minutes Cook Time: 35-45 Minutes Makes: 6 Servings

Wet Ingredients:

- 8-10 ounces (250gr) of pumpkin puree
- 2-3 eggs
- 3/4 cup vegetable oil
- ½ cup stevia

Dry Ingredients:

- 2 cups almond flour
- 1 teaspoon baking soda
- Pinch of salt
- Pinch of cinnamon
- 2 teaspoons pumpkin pie spice

Directions:

1. Start by preheating the air fryer to 330 ° F (165°C). Add the wet ingredients to a bowl and mix them. Add the dry ingredients to another bowl and mix them. Once mixed, slowly combine the dry ingredients with the wet ingredients till a batter is formed.
2. Optionally add ½ cup dried cranberries or chocolates and fold it in. Grease the inside of four pans with oil and equally divide the batter in each ramekin.
3. Place the pans in the air fryer basket and cook them for 35 to 45 minutes at 350°F (180°C). When done, take the pan out and let it rest before serving.

Per serving:

Calories 330 | Total Fat 33.6g 43% | Total Carbohydrate 5.6g 2% | Dietary Fiber 2.2g 8% | Protein 4.3g

Chewy Coconut Biscuits

Prep: 20 Minutes | Cook Time: 10-12 Minutes | Makes: 2 Servings

Ingredients:

- ½ teaspoon baking soda
- 2 tablespoons of water, boiling
- ½ cup almond flour
- ½ cup coconut flour
- ¼ cup stevia
- 1/3 cup coconut flakes
- ½ cup of organic butter

Directions:

1. Mix baking soda with boiling water and add to a large bowl. Mix the almond flour, coconut flour, stevia, coconut flakes, and butter in a baking soda bowl and mix well. Make small balls from the mixture.
2. Flat the balls in the air fryer basket. Bake for 10-12 minutes at 350°F (180°C). Once done, let it rest and then serve.

Per serving:

Calories 367 | Total Fat 40.4g 52% | Total Carbohydrate 1.8g 1% | Dietary Fiber 1g 4% | Protein 1.4g

Super Moist Cupcake

Prep: 10 Minutes | Cook Time: 15 Minutes | Makes: 4 Servings

Ingredients:

- 2 eggs
- ½ cup stevia
- ½ cup almond milk
- 1 teaspoon pure vanilla extract
- 1 cup almond flour
- ½ cup cocoa powder
- ½ teaspoon baking powder
- ¼teaspoon baking soda
- ¼teaspoon salt
- ½ cups coconut oil

Directions:

1. Crack the eggs in a bowl and add the stevia to it. Then add the almond milk and vanilla extract to the egg mixture. Take a bowl and mix the remaining dry ingredients. Add oil at the end. Now add the ingredients to the egg mixture. Then add oil to the batter. Mix it well.
2. Fill the mixture in the aluminum cupcake tray. Keep the cupcake tray in the air fryer. Bake the cupcake for 15 minutes at 350°F (180°C).
3. Once ready, take it out from the air fryer basket and serve.

Per serving:

Calories 403 | Total Fat 41.1g 54% | Total Carbohydrate 9.6g 4% | Dietary Fiber 4.7g 17% | Protein 7g

Coconut Cookies

Prep: 25 Minutes | Cook Time 8 Minutes | Makes: 4 Servings

Ingredients:

- 4-6 egg whites
- 4 teaspoons stevia
- 1 teaspoon vanilla essence
- Pinch of baking soda
- 1 cup coconut flakes, shredded coconut

Directions:

1. Preheat the air fryer before cooking to 400 ° F (205°C) for 5 minutes. Add egg whites in a bowl and use a hand beater to whisk until a stiff peak forms on opts. Add stevia and mix it again. Then add vanilla essence. Mix it well, add baking soda, and fold in coconut flakes just enough to make it a chewy and a bit lumpy batter.
2. Drop batter with a tablespoon onto an air fryer basket lined with parchment paper. Air fry for 8 minutes at 320 ° F (160°C). Once done, serve

Per serving:

Calories 91 | Total Fat 6.7g 9% | Total Carbohydrate 3.4g 1% | Dietary Fiber 1.8g 6% | Protein 4.3g

Strawberry Shortcake

Prep: 15 Minutes | Cook Time: 8-9 Minutes | Makes: 6 Servings

Strawberry Toppings:

- 2 cups sliced strawberries
- ½ cup stevia

Shortcake Ingredients:

- ¼ cup butter cold, cubed
- 2 cups Carb quick
- ½ cup stevia
- Pinch salt
- 2/3 cup water
- Garnish: sugar-free whipped cream

Directions:

1. Start by mixing strawberries with ½ cup of sweetener. Smash the strawberries using the side of the bowl and mix them. In another bowl, add butter and car quickly and mix them. Then mix stevia and salt and add water till dough is formed.
2. Divide the dough into 6 equal portions (biscuits) and arrange them in the air fryer, cooking it for 8 to 9 minutes at around 400°F (205°C).. When done, take them out and let them rest for at least 3 minutes before serving. Drizzle strawberries on top and serve with garnish.

Per serving:

Calories 211|Total Fat 15.6g 20%|Total Carbohydrate 27.6g 10%|Dietary Fiber 19.8g 71%|Protein 8.2g

Chocolate Cake

Prep: 25 Minutes | Cook Time: 25 Minutes | Makes: 4 Servings

Ingredients:

- 1.5 cups of almond flour
- ½ cup stevia
- 1/3 cup unsweetened cocoa powder
- 1/3 cup unsweetened almond milk
- 3 small eggs
- 1 teaspoon vanilla extract
- 1 teaspoon baking soda
- 1/6 teaspoon of salt

Directions:

1. Take a mixing bowl and attach paddles to it. Turn it on at low speed and mix all the above ingredients gradually by adding them.
2. Once the cake batter is ready, transfer the cake batter to a spring form pan that easily fits inside the air fryer basket.
3. Air fry the cake at 350 ° F (180°C) for 25 minutes. Once it's done, serve.

Per serving:

Calories 122 | Total Fat 9.3g 12% | Total Carbohydrate 6.7g 2% | Dietary Fiber 3.6g 13% |Protein 7.2g

Lemon Biscuits

Prep: 20 Minutes | Cook Time: 8-12 Minutes | Makes: 4 Servings

Ingredients:

- ½ cup of stevia
- 2 cups of almond flour
- ¼cup of melted butter
- 1 small lemon, zest, and juice
- 2 organic eggs
- Oil spray for greasing

Directions:

1. Preheat the Air Fryer before cooking to 400°F (205°C) for 5 minutes. Combine all the dry ingredients in a large bowl. In a separate bowl, combine all the wet ingredients.
2. Combine dry ingredients with wet ones. Mix well for good incorporation.
3. Make the dough and then roll out the dough on a flat surface. And cut your favorite shape of biscuits. Add the biscuits to an oil-greased basket.
4. Air fry it for 8-12 minutes at 350 ° F (180°C), and it does not flip. Take it out and let it cool. Serve it once done.

Per serving:

Calories 214 | Total Fat 20.8g 27% | Total Carbohydrate 3.2g 1% | Dietary Fiber 1.5g 5% | Protein 5.9g

Simple Cookies

Prep: 25 Minutes | Cook Time: 7-10 Minutes | Makes: 4 Servings

Ingredients:

- 4 tablespoons coconut oil
- 1-½ cups stevia
- 1 tablespoon vanilla extract
- 2 eggs
- 1 -½ cups almond flour
- 3/4 cup arrowroot starch
- ½ cup tablespoons coconut flour
- 1 teaspoon baking soda
- Pinch of sea salt
- 1.5 cups cocoa nibs

Directions:

1. Combine the coconut oil, stevia, and vanilla in a bowl and mix it well using an electric beater. Then add eggs to it and remix it. Now, dump the dry ingredients and beat the mixture well. Fold in the cocoa nibs at the end.
2. Preheat the air fryer basket to 350 ° F (180°C) for 5 minutes before cooking. Line the basket of the air fryer with parchment paper. Divide the dough into balls and use your palm to flatten them.
3. Arrange cookies in the air fryer basket. Bake for 5-10 minutes at 350 ° F (180°C). Once done, let it rest and then serve.

Per serving:

Calories 524 | Total Fat 54.6g 70% | Total Carbohydrate 7.5g 3% | Dietary Fiber 3.6g 13% | protein 5.5g

Pecans Brownies

Prep: 10 minutes | Cook Time: 10 minutes | makes: 4 servings

Ingredients:

- ½ cup almond flour
- 5 tablespoons stevia
- ¼teaspoon baking soda
- 6 tablespoons cocoa powder, unsweetened
- 2-3 large eggs
- ½ cup of melted butter
- ½ cup pecans, chopped

Directions:

1. Preheat an air fryer before cooking to 350 ° F (180°C) for 5 minutes. Mix the almond flour, stevia, baking powder, and cocoa powder in a large bowl. Add the egg and butter to these dry ingredients and incorporate them well. Now, fold in the pecans to it.
2. Pour it into greased ramekins and bake for 8-12 minutes at 350 ° F (180°C). Once done, serve.

Per serving:

Calories 521 | Total Fat 53.3g 68% | Total Carbohydrate 10.4g 4% | Dietary Fiber 6.5g 23% | Protein 9.4g

— Blueberry Crumble —

Prep: 25 Minutes | Cook Time: 15 Minutes | Makes: 3-4 Servings

Ingredients:

- ½ cup frozen blueberries
- Oil spray for greasing
- ¼ cup plus 1 tablespoon almond flour
- 2 tablespoons stevia
- ½ teaspoon ground cinnamon
- 2 tablespoons butter

Toppings

- 1 cup cream

Directions:

1. Preheat the air fryer before cooking to 350 ° F (180°C) for 5 minutes. Place the frozen blueberries in the bottom of a pan greased with oil spray. Combine the almond flour, stevia, cinnamon, and butter in a bowl. Mix it well so that the ingredients incorporate. Add this mixture onto the top of the blueberries Air fries it at 350 ° F (180°C) for 15 minutes. Serve and enjoy with cream as a topping.

Per serving:

Calories 104 | Total Fat 8.2g 11% | Total Carbohydrate 7g 3% | Dietary Fiber 1g 4% | Protein 1.8g

— Almond Butter Cookies —

Prep: 10 Minutes | Cook Time: 8-12 Minutes | Makes: 3-4 Servings

Ingredients:

- 1.5 cups of almond butter
- ½ cup stevia
- 4 egg whites
- ¼ teaspoon of baking soda
- 2 cups pine nuts

Directions:

1. Combine the almond butter and stevia in a bowl using a hand mixer. Then add the egg whites and baking soda. Then remix it very well. Make the dough out of this mixture.
2. Make small balls out of the dough. Roll the balls in the pine nuts and flat into cookies with a hand
3. Arrange the balls into an air fryer basket lined with parchment paper. Air fry it at 350 ° F (180°C) for 8-12 minutes, flipping halfway through. Serve and enjoy.

Per serving:

Calories 512 | Total Fat 49.9g 64% | Total Carbohydrate 10.3g 4% | Dietary Fiber 3.1g 11% | Protein 14.2g

— Apple Cider Vinegar Donuts —

Prep: 15 Minutes | Cook Time: 10 Minutes | Makes: 4 Servings

Ingredients:

- Oil spray
- 4 large eggs
- Pinch salt
- 6 teaspoons of stevia
- 2/3 cup apple cider vinegar
- 4 tablespoons coconut oil melted
- 1 teaspoon cinnamon
- 1 teaspoon baking soda
- 1 cup coconut flour

For the Drizzle:

- Turmeric Pumpkin Spice Coffee Syrup, no sugar

Directions:

1. Preheating the air fryer to around 350°F (180°C) and grease a pan with oil spray. Crack and whisk eggs, salt, stevia, apple cider vinegar, and coconut oil in a bowl.
2. In another bowl, mix cinnamon, baking soda, and coconut flour. Add the dry ingredients mixture to the wet ingredients bowl and whisk them till a batter is formed. Add the batter to the greased baking dish and make cavities in each of them.
3. Place the dish in the air fryer and cook it for 10 minutes at around 350 ° F (180°C). When done, take it out of the air fryer and place it over a wire rack, letting it cool down for 5 to 10 minutes. Drizzle pumpkin spice coffee syrupy and serve.

Per serving:

Calories 415|Total Fat 38.6g 49%|Total Carbohydrate 5.4g 2%|Dietary Fiber 2.9g 10%|Protein 13.8g

Conclusion

This keto air fryer cookbook is a treasure trove of mouthwatering and healthy recipes that are perfect for anyone, especially those following a low-carb diet or who want to follow it. With 500 recipes to choose from, there is something for all kinds of tastes and occasions. The convenience of the air fryer makes it easy to prepare these meals quickly and efficiently, so you can enjoy delicious, keto-friendly dishes without all the hassle and spending hours in the kitchen.

The wide variety of recipes ensures you will not get bored with the same old meals, and the simple directions make them easy to follow, even if you're new to the keto diet. Whether you're looking for breakfast dishes, snacks, main courses, or desserts, this cookbook has something for you.

With 500 recipes, you'll always have meal ideas and will be able to easily stay on track with your keto journey.

I hope that this book brings you a lot of pleasant emotions and that you achieve your desired results.

Appendix 1

Measurement Conversion Chart

Volume: Liquid Conversion

Metric	Imperial	USA
250 ml	8 fl ounce	1 cup
150 ml	5 fl ounce	2/3 cup
120 ml	4 fl ounce	½ cup
75 ml	2 ½ fl ounce	1/3 cup
60 ml	2 fl ounce	¼ cup
15 ml	½ fl ounce	1 tablespoon
180 ml	6 fl ounce	3/4 cup

Weight Conversion

½ ounce	15 grams
2 ounce	60 grams
4 ounce	110 grams
5 ounce	140 grams
6 ounce	170 grams
7 ounce	200 grams
8 ounce	225 grams
9 ounce	255 grams
10 ounce	280 grams
11 ounce	310 grams
12 ounce	340 grams
13 ounce	370 grams
14 ounce	400 grams
15 ounce	425 grams
1 pound	450 grams

Spoons

1 tablespoon	1/16 cup
2 tablespoons	1/8 cup
10 tablespoons	2/3 cup
4 tablespoons	¼cup
5 tablespoons	1/3 cup
8 tablespoons	½ cup
12 tablespoons	3/4 cup
16 tablespoons	1 cup

Almond Flour Conversion

USA	Metric	Imperial
1 tablespoon	6 grams	.2 ounces
¼US cup	24 grams	.8 ounces
1/3 US cup	32 grams	1.1 ounces
1/3 US cup	32 grams	1.1 ounces
1/3 US cup	32 grams	1.1 ounces

Butter

USA	Metric	Imperial
1 cup	227 grams	8 ounce
½ cup	113 grams	4 ounce
1/3 cup	75 grams	2.7 ounce
¼cup	57 grams	2 ounce

Appendix 2

Air Fryer Cooking Chart

t's important to note that the listed cooking times are approximate and can vary based on the portion size and the thickness of the food and your air fryer's specific cooking characteristics. Adjust the cooking time or temperature slightly and accordingly to achieve the desired results.

FOOD	TEMP	TIME
Brownies	325°F	40-45 Minutes
Cookies	325°F	8-10 Minutes
Cupcakes	325°F	11-13 Minutes
Mozzarella Sticks	400°F	6-8 Minutes
Veggies Fries	400°F	10-20 Minutes
Pickles	400°F	14-20 Minutes
Zucchini	400°F	12 Minutes
Asparagus	375°F	4-6 Minutes
Pork Chops	375°F	12-15 Minutes
Broccoli	400°F	8-10 Minutes
Brussels Sprouts	350°F	15-18 Minutes
Butternut Squash (Cubed)	375°F	20-25 Minutes
Carrots	375°F	15-25 Minutes
Salmon	400°F	5-7 Minutes
Sausage Patties	400°F	8-10 Minutes
Shrimp	375°F	8 Minutes
Steak	400°F	7-14 Minutes
Tilapia	400°F	6-8 Minutes
Salmon	400°F	5-7 Minutes
Chicken Breast	375°F	22-23 Minutes
Chicken Tenders	400°F	14-16 Minutes
Chicken Thighs	400°F	25 Minutes
Chicken Wings	375°F	10-12 Minutes
Bacon	400°F	5-10 Minutes
Bone-In Pork Chops	400°F	4-5 Minutes Per Side

Index

Printed in Great Britain
by Amazon

43175593R00066